Chest Wall Surgery

Guest Editor

GAETANO ROCCO, MD, FRCSEd, FETCS, FCCP

THORACIC SURGERY CLINICS

www.thoracic.theclinics.com

Consulting Editor
MARK K. FERGUSON, MD

November 2010 • Volume 20 • Number 4

SAUNDERS an imprint of ELSEVIER, Inc.

W.B. SAUNDERS COMPANY
A Division of Elsevier Inc.

1600 John F. Kennedy Boulevard • Suite 1800 • Philadelphia, Pennsylvania 19103-2899

http://www.theclinics.com

THORACIC SURGERY CLINICS Volume 20, Number 4
November 2010 ISSN 1547-4127, ISBN-13: 978-1-4377-2724-1

Editor: Catherine Bewick
Developmental Editor: Donald Mumford

Thoracic Surgery Clinics (ISSN 1547-4127) is published quarterly by Elsevier Inc., 360 Park Avenue South, New York, NY 10010-1710. Months of publication are February, May, August, and November. Business and editorial offices: 1600 John F. Kennedy Boulevard, Suite 1800, Philadelphia, PA 19103-2899. Periodicals postage paid at New York, NY, and additional mailing offices. Subscription prices are $295.00 per year (US individuals), $385.00 per year (US institutions), $141.00 per year (US Students), $367.00 per year (Canadian individuals), $487.00 per year (Canadian institutions), $192.00 per year (Canadian and foreign students), $391.00 per year (foreign individuals), and $487.00 per year (foreign institutions). Foreign air speed delivery is included in all Clinics' subscription prices. All prices are subject to change without notice. **POSTMASTER:** Send address changes to Thoracic Surgery Clinics, Elsevier Health Sciences Division, Subscription Customer Service, 3251 Riverport Lane, Maryland Heights, MO 63043. **Customer Service (orders, claims, online, change of address): Telephone: 1-800-654-2452 (U.S. and Canada); 314-447-8871 (outside U.S. and Canada). Fax: 314-447-8029. Email: journalscustomerservice-usa@elsevier.com (for print support); journalsonlinesupport-usa@elsevier.com (for online support).**

Reprints. For copies of 100 or more, of articles in this publication, please contact Commercial Rights Department, Elsevier Inc., 360 Park Avenue South, New York, NY 10010-1710. Tel: (212) 633-3812; Fax: (212) 462-1935; E-mail: reprints@elsevier.com.

Thoracic Surgery Clinics is covered in *MEDLINE/PubMed (Index Medicus)* and *EMBASE/Excerpta Medica.*

Printed and bound by CPI Group (UK) Ltd, Croydon, CR0 4YY

Transferred to Digital Print 2012

Contributors

CONSULTING EDITOR

MARK K. FERGUSON, MD
Professor of Surgery, Section of Cardiac
and Thoracic Surgery, The University of
Chicago Medical Center, Chicago, Illinois

GUEST EDITOR

**GAETANO ROCCO, MD, FRCSEd,
FETCS, FCCP**
Director, Department of Thoracic
Surgery and Oncology,
Chief, Division of Thoracic Surgery,
National Cancer Institute, Pascale Foundation,
Naples, Italy

AUTHORS

ALEX ARAME, MD
Department of Thoracic Surgery,
Georges Pompidou European Hospital,
Paris, France

JUSTIN D. BLASBERG, MD
Resident, Department of General Surgery,
St Luke's—Roosevelt Medical Center,
Columbia University College of Physicians
and Surgeons, New York, New York

LAURENT BROUCHET, MD, PhD
Department of Thoracic Surgery,
Rangueil-Larrey University Hospital,
Toulouse, France

DAVID W. CHANG, MD, FACS
Professor, Department of Plastic Surgery,
University of Texas MD Anderson Cancer
Center, Houston, Texas

ALAIN CHAPELIER, MD, PhD
Professor of Thoracic and Cardiovascular
Surgery, Paris West University; Head,
Department of Thoracic Surgery and Lung
Transplantation, Hôpital Foch, Suresnes,
France

MARCELLINO CICALESE, MD
Division of Breast Surgery, Department
of Breast Surgery and Oncology, National
Cancer Institute of Naples, Naples, Italy

SABRINA CUGNO, MD
Senior Resident, Division of Plastic and
Reconstructive Surgery, Department of
Surgery, Centre Hospitalier de l'Universite
de Montreal, Universite de Montreal,
Montreal, Quebec, Canada

GIUSEPPE D'AIUTO, MD
Division of Thoracic Surgery, Department
of Thoracic Surgery and Oncology, National
Cancer Institute of Naples, Naples, Italy

MASSIMILIANO D'AIUTO, MD
Division of Thoracic Surgery, Department of
Thoracic Surgery and Oncology, National
Cancer Institute of Naples, Naples, Italy

MICHEL ALAIN DANINO, MD, PhD
Associate Professor of Surgery, Division
of Plastic and Reconstructive Surgery,
Department of Surgery, Centre Hospitalier
de l'Universite de Montreal, Universite de
Montreal, Montreal, Quebec, Canada

JESSICA S. DONINGTON, MD
Assistant Professor, Department
of Cardiothoracic Surgery, NYU School
of Medicine; Director of Thoracic Surgery,
Department of Cardiothoracic Surgery,
Bellevue Hospital, New York, New York

PASQUALE FERRARO, MD
Associate Professor of Surgery, Chief,
Division of Thoracic Surgery; Alfonso
Minicozzi and Family Chair in Thoracic
Surgery and Lung Transplantation,
Department of Surgery, Centre Hospitalier
de l'Universite de Montreal, Universite de
Montreal, Montreal, Quebec, Canada

ALEXANDER A. FOKIN, MD, PhD
Heineman Medical Research Foundation,
Charlotte, North Carolina

SHAF KESHAVJEE, MD, MSc, FRCSC, FACS
Surgeon-In-Chief, University Health Network;
FG Pearson-RJ Ginsberg Chair in Thoracic
Surgery; Professor and Chair, Division of
Thoracic Surgery, University of Toronto,
Toronto General Hospital, Toronto, Ontario,
Canada

PATRICK G. HARRIS, MD CM
Associate Professor, Chair, Department of
Surgery, Centre Hospitalier de l'Universite
de Montreal, Universite de Montreal,
Montreal, Quebec, Canada

ROBERT E. KELLY Jr, MD
Chief, Department of Surgery, Children's
Hospital of The King's Daughters;
Professor of Clinical Surgery and
Pediatrics, Eastern Virginia Medical
School, Norfolk, Virginia

FRANÇOISE LE PIMPEC BARTHES, MD, PhD
Department of Thoracic Surgery, Georges
Pompidou European Hospital, Paris, France

MOISHE LIBERMAN, MD CM, PhD
Assistant Professor of Surgery, Marcel and
Rolande Gosselin Chair in Thoracic Surgical
Oncology, Division of Thoracic Surgery,
Department of Surgery, Centre Hospitalier de
l'Universite de Montreal, Universite de
Montreal, Montreal, Quebec, Canada

TAMAS F. MOLNAR, MD, PhD
Professor, Department of Surgery, Thoracic
Surgical Unit, University of Pécs, Pécs,
Hungary

BABU V. NAIDU, MBBS
(MMed Sci Trauma) MD, FRCS (CTH)
Associate Professor, Heart of England NHS
Foundation Trust, Department of Thoracic
Surgery, Birmingham; Warwick Medical
School, The University of Warwick, Coventry,
United Kingdom

DONALD NUSS, MB, ChB
Professor of Surgery and Pediatrics,
Pediatric Surgery, Eastern Virginia Medical
School, Children's Hospital of The King's
Daughters, Norfolk, Virginia

JOE B. PUTNAM Jr, MD
Professor of Surgery and Chairman,
Department of Thoracic Surgery; Ingram
Professor of Cancer Research, Professor
of Biomedical Informatics, Vanderbilt
University Medical Center, Nashville,
Tennessee

PALA B. RAJESH, MBBS, FRCS (CTH)
Honorary Senior Lecturer, Heart of England
NHS Foundation Trust, Department
of Thoracic Surgery, Birmingham,
United Kingdom

MARC RIQUET, MD, PhD
Department of Thoracic Surgery,
Georges Pompidou European Hospital,
Paris, France

FRANCIS ROBICSEK, MD, PhD
Department of Thoracic and Cardiovascular
Surgery, Sanger Heart and Vascular Institute,
Carolinas Medical Center, Charlotte,
North Carolina

GAETANO ROCCO, MD, FRCSEd,
FETCS, FCCP
Director, Department of Thoracic
Surgery and Oncology,
Chief, Division of Thoracic Surgery,
National Cancer Institute, Pascale Foundation,
Naples, Italy

SHONA E. SMITH, MD, FRCSC
Thoracic Surgery Fellow, Division
of Thoracic Surgery, University
of Toronto, Toronto General Hospital,
Toronto, Ontario, Canada

PASCAL A. THOMAS, MD
Department of Thoracic Surgery,
University Hospitals of Marseille,
University of the Mediterranean, Marseille,
France

MARK T. VILLA, MD
Assistant Professor, Department of Plastic
Surgery, University of Texas MD Anderson
Cancer Center, Houston, Texas

LARRY T. WATTS, MD
Department of Thoracic and Cardiovascular
Surgery, Sanger Heart and Vascular Institute,
Carolinas Medical Center, Charlotte,
North Carolina

Contents

> The chest wall, like other regional anatomy, is a remarkable fusion of form and function. Principal functions are the protection of internal viscera and an expandable cylinder facilitating variable gas flow into the lungs. Knowledge of the anatomy of the whole cylinder (ribs, sternum, vertebra, diaphragm, intercostal spaces, and extrathoracic muscles) is therefore not only important in the local environment of a specific chest wall resection but also in its relation to overall function. An understanding of chest wall kinematics might help define the loss of function after resection and the effects of various chest wall substitutes. Therefore, this article is not an exhaustive anatomic description but a focused summary and discussion.

> Despite significant improvements in surgical technique and perioperative care, the management of patients requiring chest wall resection and reconstruction is an ongoing challenge for thoracic surgeons. A successful approach includes a thorough assessment of the patient and the lesion, an adequate biopsy to confirm tissue diagnosis, and a well-established treatment plan. In the case of a primary tumor of the chest wall, the extent of the resection should not be limited by the size of the resulting defect. Following resection, chest wall reconstruction mandates an appreciation for restoration of functional and structural components. An algorithmic approach to chest wall reconstruction begins with the assessment of the nature of the defect, taking into consideration factors such as infection, tumor location, previous radiation therapy, and surgical intervention. The latter factors bear influence on the type of tissue required as well as whether reconstruction can be performed in a single stage or whether it is better delayed. Finally, patient factors including lifestyle and work, as well as prognosis, are considered to determine the best reconstructive option.

> Recent paradigm shift in major trauma profile elevates chest wall injuries among the most important topics of the specialty. Due to mass casualties of terror attacks and asymmetric warfare, civilian and military trauma care challenges thoracic surgery, traumatology, intensive anesthesiology, and related specialties. Contemporary advances of the main issues are systemically presented and discussed, such as soft tissue and bony structure injuries, complex traumas like flail chest, and extensively destroyed chest wall.

> Soft tissue necrosis secondary to infection and radiation injury account for the majority of chest wall resections performed today that are unrelated to malignancy.

Principles of treatment for chest wall infection and necrosis rely partially on the underlying cause and overall health of the patient but, in general, are based on wide resection of devitalized tissue and subsequent reconstruction with soft tissue coverage. Unlike resection for malignancy, fibrosis of underlying tissues often precludes skeletal reconstruction without concurrent loss of chest wall integrity or pulmonary function. Although the surgical intervention of these processes is similar, the underlying pathology differs significantly. This article addresses the risk factors, pathophysiology, clinical presentation, and management of chest wall and sterno-clavicular joint infections, necrotizing processes, and radiation injury.

The differential diagnosis of chest wall tumors is diverse, including both benign and malignant lesions (primary and malignant), local extension of adjacent disease, and local manifestations of infectious and inflammatory processes. Primary chest wall tumors are best classified by their primary component: soft tissue or bone. Work-up consists of a thorough history, physical examination and imaging to best assess location, size, composition, association with surrounding structures, and evidence of any soft tissue component. Biopsies are often required, especially for soft tissue masses. Treatment depends on histological subtype and location, but may include chemotherapy and radiotherapy in addition to surgical resection.

Chest wall involvement by breast cancer remains a difficult clinical challenge that may occur at the time of the primary diagnosis or later as a result of locoregional breast cancer recurrence. A case-by-case multidisciplinary approach is strongly recommended, and a multimodality therapy should be always considered. Full-thickness resection of the chest wall can be done with acceptable morbidity and mortality, providing a good palliation and a better quality of life even to patients with poor prognosis. Moreover, in well-selected cases, chest wall resection results in locoregional control of disease and prolongation of life.

Non–Small cell lung cancer invading the chest wall represents an advanced stage of the disease. Chest wall resection may be achieved in up to 100% of the patients, and the ensuing defect requires to be reconstructed in 40% to 64% of cases. Once a sur-gical challenge, chest wall resection is no longer a technical problem and en bloc chest wall and lung resections regularly provide good results. However, survival rates are jeopardized by incompleteness of the resection and mediastinal lymph node involvement. Nowadays, the challenge is represented by the use of the other nonsurgical modalities (chemotherapy and radiation therapy) to increase the chance of performing a complete resection, the need to achieve a better control of probable lymphatic or hematogenous spread, and the reduction of the recurrence rate.

Radical resection can offer a definitive cure of primary malignant sternal tumors, but the surgical management may be difficult because of the local aggressiveness of

these tumors and a high recurrence rate. This article describes improvements in reconstruction techniques with musculocutaneous flaps that have made coverage of
wide sternal defects reliable. A rigid reinforcement of the sternum can now be
achieved with titanium bars and clips after a total sternectomy. Large sternal defects
are safely reconstructed with a musculocutaneous flap. The completeness of the resection and the histologic grade of the tumors are the strongest survival predictors.

Chest wall resection requires wide local excision, negative margins, and adequate
reconstruction. Outcomes are generally good to excellent with wide local excision
and negative margins. Mortality is nearly 0% to 1% with mild morbidity. Multispecialty surgical teams may be required for more complex situations. Early diagnosis of
chest wall sarcomas, confirmation by an experienced sarcoma pathologist, and multidisciplinary discussion before treatment initiation, are all required for optimal and
successful therapy.

Reconstruction of the chest wall represents an important part of a patient's treatment following resection of various thoracic tumors. Many different types of flaps,
including both pedicled and free flaps, have been described for use in chest wall reconstruction. These reconstructions are most effectively managed with a multidisciplinary approach involving plastic and cardiothoracic surgery. The pectoralis major,
latissimus dorsi, rectus abdominis, trapezius, and external oblique muscles and the
omentum are all local options that can play an important role in the reconstruction of
the chest wall.

Chest wall reconstructions can be complex and challenging procedures, especially
when huge thoracic defects have been generated by radical excisions. Nonrigid reconstructions with meshes or patches have the goal of avoiding a lung hernia
caused by the chest wall defect, or preventing the impaction of the scapula in
case of posterior chest wall resections, especially when the resection is extended
down to the 5th and 6th ribs. Large anterior and lateral resections result in thoracic
instability and alteration of pulmonary physiology, and render intrathoracic structures vulnerable to external impact. They necessitate rigid reconstructions according to several techniques using alloplastic materials (eg, methyl methacrylate-based
customized plates or neo-ribs, osteosynthesis systems, or dedicated prosthesis).
Nowadays, the availability of these multiple, possibly combined, more adapted,
and better tolerated materials have pushed past the limits of resection to those involving soft tissue coverage.

This article focuses on new materials available to thoracic surgeons for the reconstruction of chest wall defects. Each surgeon is called to select the best reconstructive strategy based on the disease for which the resection is needed, the possible

extension to adjacent structures, the availability of professional colleagues for multidisciplinary involvement, and the preferred (or available) material for full or partial thickness reconstruction.

Pectus Carinatum   563

Francis Robicsek and Larry T. Watts

Pectus carinatum or keel chest is a spectrum of progressive inborn anomalies of the anterior chest wall, named after the keel (carina) of ancient Roman ships. It defines a wide spectrum of inborn protrusion anomalies of the sternum and/or the adjacent costal cartilages. Pectus carinatum is often associated with various conditions, notably Marfan disease, homocystinuria, prune belly, Morquio syndrome, osteogenesis imperfecta, Noonan syndrome, and mitral valve prolapse. Treatment of pectus carinatum by nonsurgical methods such as exercise and casting has not been worthwhile, whereas surgical management is simple and successful.

Thoracic Defects: Cleft Sternum and Poland Syndrome   575

Alexander A. Fokin

Defects of the thoracic cage with bone and/or muscle deficit are relatively rare and can present a real risk depending on the severity of manifestations. Cleft sternum results from failed midline fusion of the sternal halves that leaves the heart and great vessels unprotected, and is commonly associated with craniofacial hemangiomas. Correction is recommended during the neonatal period when compliant thorax allows direct suturing of the divided sternum. Sternal foramen requires precaution during biopsy and acupuncture as well as forensic awareness. In addition to the thoracic defect, Poland syndrome can be associated with hand anomalies, dextrocardia, renal agenesia, and various tumors. Age and gender, together with the degree of the defect, define the method of surgical correction.

Indications and Technique of Nuss Procedure for Pectus Excavatum   583

Donald Nuss and Robert E. Kelly Jr

Pectus excavatum most frequently involves the lower sternum and chest wall. Because the morphology varies, preoperative imaging for anatomic assessment and documentation of dimensions of the chest are important. Many modifications have been made to the minimally invasive procedure since it was first performed in 1987. As a result, there has been an increase in the number of patients seeking surgical correction. This article discusses the clinical features of pectus excavatum and reviews the preoperative considerations and the steps involved in the repair of the deformity.

Index   599

Thoracic Surgery Clinics

THE CLINICS ARE NOW AVAILABLE ONLINE!

Access your subscription at:
www.theclinics.com

Preface

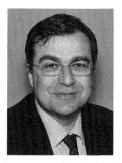

Gaetano Rocco, MD, FRCSEd, FETCS, FCCP
Guest Editor

This issue of *Thoracic Surgery Clinics* is dedicated to a technical aspect of the clinical practice with which surgeons have become increasingly familiar through the years. Indeed, by the term "chest wall surgery," a wide variety of procedures are referred to, varying from a straightforward removal of one rib or the correction of a congenital malformation to an extremely complex resection and subsequent reconstruction of the chest wall primarily aimed at preserving geometric and functional integrity. As such, chest wall surgery can offer scenarios where the creativity and the technical skills are emphasized to an unprecedented level in the thoracic surgical practice.

The introduction of new biomaterials or the proposal of time-honored ones made of different alloys designed for the chest wall have made it possible to perform previously unimaginable resections with excellent functional, oncologic, and cosmetic results. The field of chest wall surgery has also become the ideal setting for multidisciplinary collaboration between thoracic surgeons and their orthopedic, plastic, and neurosurgical colleagues aimed at identifying the best solution for an often challenging situation such as posttraumatic stabilization, radiation injuries, and primary and secondary chest wall tumors, with particular attention to primary sarcomas and to the chest wall infiltration from lung tumors and the complication of breast cancer treatment. The basic anatomic and functional tenets of chest wall surgery, together with a current view of the available materials for chest wall reconstruction, are outlined, without forgetting a glimpse into the possible future. Finally, a comprehensive review of the indications and the technical challenges in the correction of chest wall malformations is provided to complete the overview of a surgical discipline where the combination of technological advancements and outstanding manual dexterity, along with an improved understanding of the topographical details of the human anatomy, is producing one of the most gratifying domains in our profession.

Gaetano Rocco, MD, FRCSEd, FETCS, FCCP
Department of Thoracic Surgery and Oncology
Division of Thoracic Surgery
National Cancer Institute, Pascale Foundation
Naples, Italy

E-mail address:
Gaetano.Rocco@btopenworld.com

Thorac Surg Clin 20 (2010) xiii
doi:10.1016/j.thorsurg.2010.06.007

Relevant Surgical Anatomy of the Chest Wall

Babu V. Naidu, MBBS (MMed Sci Trauma), MD, FRCS (CTH)[a,b,*],
Pala B. Rajesh, MBBS, FRCS (CTH)[a]

KEYWORDS

• Chest wall anatomy • Costal cartilage • Tubercle

SKELETAL STRUCTURES
Ribs

The ribs and costal cartilages form the lateral aspects of the thoracic cylinder.[1] Ribs have a head, a neck, a tubercle, an articular facet, and a shaft (**Fig. 1**).

The first 7 are "true ribs" because they articulate posteriorly with the vertebrae and anteriorly with the sternum by means of a costal cartilage and a true synovial joint. The flat short broad first rib and the little larger second rib do not contribute in a major fashion to thoracic volume increase in enhanced ventilation because of their size and their limited range of motion.

The last 5 are "false ribs," either because they articulate anteriorly with the seventh costal cartilage (ribs 8–10) or because their anterior extremity ends freely in the posterolateral abdominal wall ("floating ribs," 11 and 12) (**Fig. 2**).

The posterior rib head presents an articular surface with 2 facets per head, divided by a crest, for articulation with its 2 adjacent vertebrae. The lower facet articulates with the superior articular facet of the numerically corresponding vertebral body (see **Fig. 1**). Exceptions are the first, 11th, and 12th rib in which there is a single articular facet.

The neck of the rib spans between the head and the tubercle. The tubercle is the posterior bulging of the rib that articulates with the transverse process of the similarly numbered vertebra (see **Fig. 1**). The inferior costal groove of the rib forms just beyond the tubercle and protects the intercostal neurovascular bundle.

The breadth of the intercostal spaces is greater anteriorly than posteriorly, and greater between the upper ribs than the lower ribs.

Sternum

The sternum consists of 3 bony parts connected by 2 joints. The wide cephalad manubrium is relatively fixed because it articulates with the first rib and the clavicle. The large flat body of the sternum articulates with ribs 2 through 7 (**Fig. 3**). The joint between the manubrium and the body moves allowing the body to move anteriorly and cephalad. In the process it draws the ribs, which articulate with it, upward and outward, increasing the transverse diameter of the chest. The xiphoid process is small and is of little consequence.

Thoracic Vertebrae

On the posterolateral aspect of each thoracic vertebral body are found 2 articular surfaces, the superior and inferior costal articular facets of the thoracic vertebra (**Fig. 4**). The superior costal articular facet lies just anterior to the arch pedicle.

The transverse process projects posterolaterally and slightly upward from the area in which the arch pedicle joins the lamina. The transverse process articular facet sits on its anterolateral aspect, near its distal tip. The 11th and 12th thoracic

[a] Heart of England NHS Foundation Trust, Department of Thoracic Surgery, Bordesley Green East, Birmingham, B9 5SS, UK
[b] Warwick Medical School, The University of Warwick, Gibbet Hill Road, Coventry, CV4 7AL, UK
* Corresponding author. Heart of England NHS Foundation Trust, Department of Thoracic Surgery, Bordesley Green East, Birmingham, B9 5SS, UK.
E-mail address: babu.naidu@heartofengland.nhs.uk

Thorac Surg Clin 20 (2010) 453–463
doi:10.1016/j.thorsurg.2010.07.006
1547-4127/10/$ — see front matter © 2010 Published by Elsevier Inc.

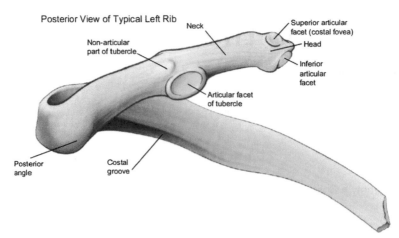

Fig. 1. An example of a true left rib showing the tubercle, the neck, and the head of the rib. The head harbors a superior and an inferior articular facet. (*From* Vallières E. The costovertebral angle. Thorac Surg Clin 2007; 17(4):503–10; with permission.)

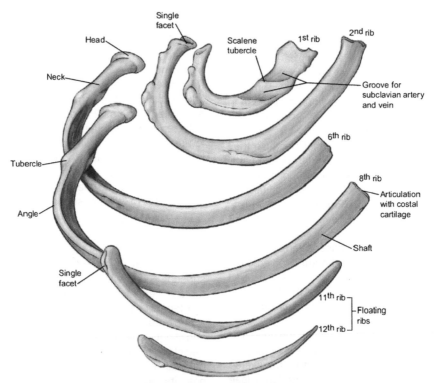

Fig. 2. The characteristics of ribs. Ribs 3 through 10, articulate with the spine posteriorly and with the sternum costal cartilages anteriorly. These are larger ribs that have greater excursion. They therefore cause a greater increase in the diameter of the chest when they are lifted cephalad and decrease the diameter correspondingly when they are drawn inferiorly by the accessory muscles of the respiration, causing forced expiration. The heads of these ribs have 2 fascicular aspects and therefore are wedge shaped. The tubercles of all these ribs consist of an articular surface and a nonarticular surface. All have well-developed costal grooves that protect the intercostal bundle consisting of the intercostal artery, the intercostal vein, and the nerve. The posterior part of the body of these ribs is rounded, and the anterior part of the body is flat. The anterior articular surface in which the rib joins the corresponding costal cartilage is cup shaped. (*From* Graeber GM, Nazim M. The anatomy of the ribs and the sternum and their relationship to chest wall structure and function. Thorac Surg Clin 2007; 17(4):473–89; with permission).

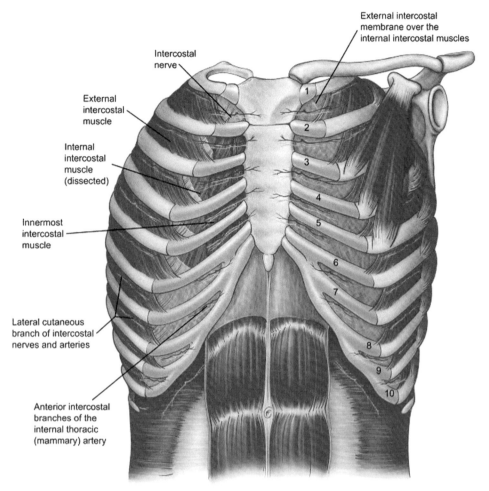

Fig. 3. Anterior chest wall showing the sternum. Note where the costal cartilages articulate with the sternum. In the intercostal space lie different structures: several kinds of intercostal muscles, intercostal arteries and associated veins, lymphatics, and nerves. (*From* Rendina EA, Ciccone AM. The intercostal space. Thorac Surg Clin 2007;17(4):491–501; with permission.)

vertebrae usually have a single superior costal and no transverse process articular facet.

From the capacious thoracic intervertebral foramen, the spinal ganglion and nerve root and branches of the spinal arterial and venous systems emerge. The foramen, limited above and below by the pedicles of the 2 adjacent vertebrae lying directly in front and below, is the base of each transverse process, which is a useful surgical landmark.

The ribs are joined to the vertebral bodies by 2 articulations: one linking the head of the rib with its adjoining vertebral bodies (the costovertebral joint), and one in between the rib tubercle and the transverse process of the vertebra (the costotransverse joint).

As mentioned, costovertebral joint cavity (ribs 2–10) contains the upper facet of the rib head that is in contact with the inferior costal facet of the vertebral body above and the lower head facet

that articulates with the superior costal facet of the numerically corresponding vertebra, and is partially divided by an interarticular ligament that attaches a crest situated in between the 2 joint facets of the head and with intervertebral disk. The capsule gains much support that comes from the radiate ligament or anterior costovertebral ligament, which attaches to the rib head anteriorly and to the sides of the articulating vertebral bodies and the intervertebral disk (**Fig. 5**). A smaller ligament, the posterior costovertebral ligament, unites the rib to the anterior aspect of the corresponding intervertebral foramen above and the external aspect of the arch pedicle below.

The costotransverse joint is a small synovial cavity held together by ligaments, principally superior and posterior, which extend from the inferior aspect of the transverse process above to the superior aspect of the rib tubercle below. The

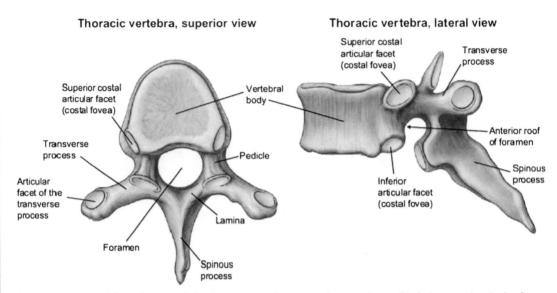

Thoracic vertebra, superior view

Thoracic vertebra, lateral view

Fig. 4. Superior and lateral views of the thoracic vertebra. Note the superior and inferior costal articular facets, which articulate with the heads of the adjacent ribs. The transverse process also presents an articular facet to join the rib tubercle. (*From* Vallières E. The costovertebral angle. Thorac Surg Clin 2007;17(4):503—10; with permission.)

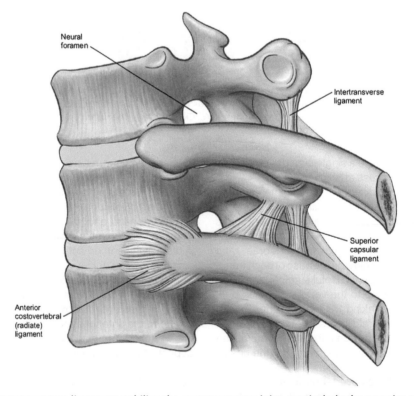

Fig. 5. The costotransverse ligaments stabilize the costotransverse joint, particularly the superior and posterior (not shown) costotransverse ligaments. (*From* Vallières E. The costovertebral angle. Thorac Surg Clin 2007; 17(4):503—10; with permission.)

dorsal ramus of the intercostal nerve root and posterior branch of the segmental artery (which gives off a branch to supply the cord) runs medial to this ligament to the paraspinal muscle mass.

MUSCULAR STRUCTURES
Intercostal Muscles

Between 12 ribs are 11 intercostal spaces that comprise intercostal muscles and membranes that supply neurovascular structures (see **Fig. 3**). External intercostal muscles extend from the rib tubercles dorsally to the costal cartilages anteriorly. Arising from the lower border of the rib above, fibers run obliquely downward, forward, and insert into the upper border of the rib below. In the upper 2 spaces they do not reach the anterior end of the ribs and in the lower 2 they become continuous with the external oblique muscles at the end of the costal cartilages. The internal intercostal muscles run further anterior to the sternum but extend only as far as the angle of the rib. Arising from the inferior border on the inner surface of the rib that lies superiorly, and from the corresponding costal cartilage, fibers run obliquely inferiorly and posteriorly and insert into the upper border of the rib below. A third layer is interposed between the 2 planes of muscular fibers and is more developed where the muscular fibers are deficient.

The innermost intercostals are variable and incomplete, and fibers run in the direction of the fibers of the internal intercostals, but they lie deep to the intercostal neurovascular bundle. The subcostalis (or infracostal) muscles, which could be considered part of this third group of muscles, vary in size and number and lie on the internal surface of the lower ribs, usually in the lower part of the thorax. The subcostalis muscles arise from the inner surface of one rib near its angle and are inserted into the inner surface of the second or third rib below.

Diaphragm

The diaphragm is an elliptical cylindroid structure, capped by a dome; it arches over the abdomen, with the right hemidiaphragm higher than the left (**Fig. 6**). The concave, dome-shaped part allows the liver and the spleen, situated underneath the diaphragm, to be protected by the lower ribs and the chest wall.

The diaphragm is a striated skeletal muscle consisting of 2 major parts: the muscular part radiating outward and the central, noncontractile tendinous part. The tripart muscular diaphragm originates from the lumbar spine (L1−3) dorsally, lower 6 ribs laterally, and xiphisternum ventrally, and have different embryologic origins, segmental innervation, and functional properties.

The lumbocostal triangles/trigones (Bochdalek gap) exist between the lumbar and costal parts of the diaphragm, more commonly on the left side than on the right side usually closed only by fascia, peritoneum, and pleura. Anteriorly, there are bilateral triangular gaps between the sternal and costal parts (named after Morgagni and Larrey, or the sternocostal triangles) through which pass the internal thoracic/superior epigastric vessels.

The highest part of the diaphragm, the central tendon, in which all the musculature of the diaphragm inserts, has a cloverleaf-like shape, and lies anteriorly attached firmly to the pericardium. Laterally, the right and left diaphragmatic dome parts are mobile, and their position depends on the extent of ventilation.

The diaphragm has an enormously rich blood supply; hence, necrosis is rare. The arterial blood supply to the diaphragm is derived from (1) the pericardiophrenic arteries running with the phrenic nerves, (2) the musculophrenic arteries, (3) the superior and inferior phrenic (main source) arteries, and (4) the intercostal arteries (peripheral). The veins of the diaphragm follow the arteries and are accompanied by lymphatic vessels. The diaphragmatic blood flow is respiratory phase dependent: it increases during the diaphragmatic relaxation and decreases during inspiration. During resistance breathing, diaphragmatic blood flow increases more than 20-fold. Diaphragmatic contractility depends on appropriate oxygen supply and so it is important that it returns to its constant resting position.[2]

The phrenic nerve supplies motor and sensory innervations and the sixth and/or seventh intercostal nerves, the latter distributed to the costal part of the diaphragm. The muscular part of the diaphragm receives its main motor innervation via the phrenic nerves originating in the cervical plexus running craniocaudally passing anterior to the hilum of the lungs, attaching to the pericardium, and on the right side pierces the central tendon anterolaterally to the vena caval opening and on the left lateral to the border of the heart and anterior to the central tendon. The phrenic nerves give branches on the thoracic side of the diaphragm: anteromedially to the sternum, anterolaterally to the costal diaphragm, and posteromedially to the crural diaphragm in a radial fashion. The diaphragm has 3 anatomic openings: the aortic, the esophageal, and the inferior vena cava orifices.

Breathing is endurance work, like that of the heart, because the diaphragm must contract in repetitive fashion for life. Hence it contains 55% type I, slow-twitch, fatigue-resistant muscle fibers; the remaining type II, fast-twitch are recruited when the breathing rate increases.[3]

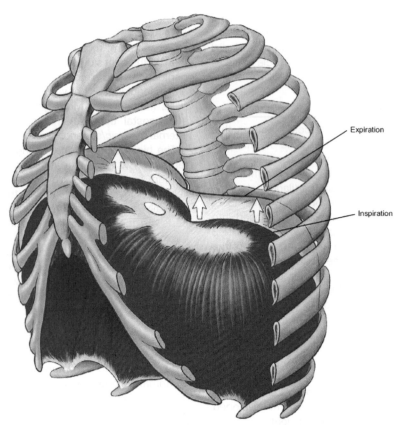

Fig. 6. The anatomic features of the diaphragm allow it to draw the central tendon downward so it performs as a piston. The radially arranged fibers originate from the skeletal structures at the base of the cylinder (including the 10th rib, the costal arches, and the sternum anteriorly) and insert on the central tendon. When the fibers are fired by the phrenic nerves, the resulting contraction draws the central tendon downward. The diaphragm in its relaxed state is dome shaped. When the muscle fibers contract, the central tendon is drawn downward, causing the diaphragm to flatten. Contraction of the diaphragm moves the abdominal viscera downward, expands the lung, and causes inspiration. (*From* Graeber GM, Nazim M. The anatomy of the ribs and the sternum and their relationship to chest wall structure and function. Thorac Surg Clin 2007;17(4):473–89; with permission.)

Extrathoracic Muscles

Knowledge of function and anatomy of extrathoracic chest wall muscles is essential to understand the effects of resection and appropriate use as muscle flaps (**Fig. 7**).[4] An overview is given in **Table 1**.

Neurovascular Structures

The intercostal neurovascular bundle lies between the internal and innermost intercostal muscles or parietal pleura in which the intercostal vein is most cephalad, followed by the artery and nerve caudally. In each intercostal space there are 2 sets of arteries, posterior and anterior, that anastomose with each other. In each space, the single posterior intercostal arteries originate from ventral branches of segmental arteries from the descending thoracic aorta, and the smaller twin anterior (coursing above and below each rib) are branches of the internal thoracic artery or its terminal branch, the musculophrenic artery. The exception is the first 2 intercostal spaces, which originate from the superior intercostal artery posteriorly (costocervical trunk) and the supreme thoracic artery (axillary artery) anteriorly. This twin blood supply has obvious advantages to proximal and distal perfusion of the chest wall after resection. The intercostal veins have a similar distribution to that of the arteries; posteriorly draining into the azygos and accessory/hemiazygos systems (except the uppermost into the brachiocephalic vein) and anteriorly into the internal thoracic veins.

After exiting the intervertebral foramen, the spinal root gives off 2 branches: the dorsal or posterior ramus, which supplies the muscles, bones, and joints of the posterior thoracic wall, and the ventral or anterior ramus, which becomes

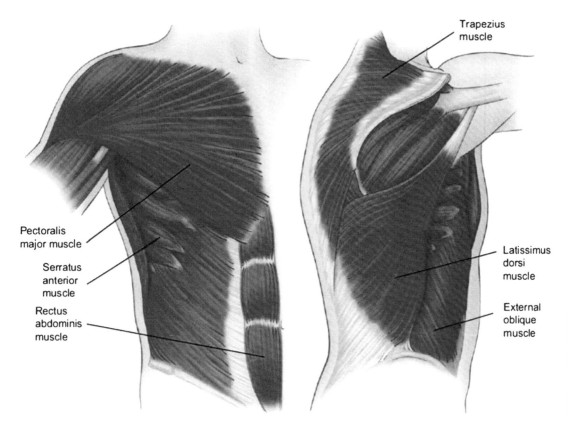

Fig. 7. Overview of chest wall and extrathoracic muscles that can be used for chest wall reconstruction. (*From* Miller JI Jr. Muscles of the chest wall. Thorac Surg Clin 2007;17(4):464–72; with permission.)

the intercostal nerve running in the subcostal groove of the rib except for the 12th, which lies below the rib and is called the subcostal nerve.

The first 2 nerves supply fibers to the upper extremities in addition to their thoracic branches; the next 4 are limited to the thorax, and the lower 5 supply thorax and upper abdomen. This structure accounts for the distribution of pain caused by chest wall infiltration. The nerves pass forward in the intercostal spaces below the intercostal vessels, initially lying between the pleura and the intercostal membranes, but soon piercing the latter and running between the 2 planes of intercostal muscles as far as the middle of the rib. The nerves then enter the substance of the internal intercostals, running amid their fibers as far as the costal cartilages, where they reach the inner surfaces of the muscles and lie between them and the pleura. Near the sternum, they cross in front of the internal mammary artery and pierce the internal intercostals, the anterior intercostal membranes, and pectoralis major, and supply the integument of the front of the thorax and over the breast, forming the anterior cutaneous branches of the thorax. At the front of the thorax

some of these branches cross the costal cartilages from one intercostal space to another. Lateral cutaneous branches derived from the intercostal nerves midway pierce the external intercostals and serratus anterior, and divide into anterior and posterior branches. The anterior branches run forward to the side and the forepart of the chest, supplying the skin and the mamma; those of the fifth and sixth nerves supply the upper digitations of the external oblique abdominis. The posterior branches run backward, and supply the skin over the scapula and latissimus dorsi. The lower thoracic nerves (7th–11th) continue anteriorly from the intercostal spaces into the abdominal wall between the internal oblique and transversus abdominis, to the sheath of the rectus abdominis, which they perforate. The lower intercostal nerves supply the intercostals and abdominal muscles; the last 3 send branches to the serratus posterior inferior.

The Intercostal Lymphatic Vessels

At the anterior ends of the intercostal spaces are the sternal glands, by the side of the internal mammary artery; the posterior parts of the

Table 1
Extra-thoracic chest wall muscles

Muscle	Origin	Insertion	Artery	Nerve	Action	Use and Consequence
Trapezius	Midline from the external occipital protuberance, nuchal ligament, medial part superior nuchal line, spinous processes vertebrae C7–T12	At the shoulders, into the lateral third of the clavicle, the acromion process and into the spine of the scapula	Transverse cervical artery	Cranial nerve XI. Cervical nerves III & IV receive information about pain	Retraction of scapula	Used for upper chest and neck defects
Latissimus dorsi	Spinous processes of thoracic T6–T12, thoracolumbar fascia, iliac crest, and inferior 3 or 4 ribs	Floor of intertubercular groove of the humerus	Subscapular artery, dorsal scapular artery	Thoracodorsal nerve	Pulls the forelimb dorsally and caudally	Lateral and anterior chest wall defect. Excellent musculocutaneous collaterals allow significant skin to be taken
Pectoralis major	Anterior surface of medial half of clavicle Sternocostal head: anterior surface of the sternum, the superior 6 costal cartilages	Intertubercular groove of the humerus	Pectoral branch thoracoacromial trunk and internal mammary, lateral intercostal arteries, and lateral thoracic perforators	Lateral and medial pectoral nerve Clavicular head: C5/6 Sternocostal head: C7/8 T1	Clavicular head: flexes the humerus Sternocostal head: extends the humerus As a whole, adducts and medially and rotates the humerus. Draws scapula anterioinferiorly	Anterior and midline (sternal defects). Used as a pedicle graft based on the primary blood supply or as a turnover flap on secondary supply. Possible displacement of the breast and abduction medial rotation loss of arm

Muscle	Origin	Insertion	Blood supply	Nerve supply	Action	Comments
Serratus anterior	Fleshy slips from the outer surface of upper 8 or 9 ribs	Costal aspect of medial margin of the scapula	Lateral thoracic artery (upper part), thoracodorsal artery (lower part)	Long thoracic nerve from roots of brachial plexus C5–C7	Protract and stabilizes scapula, assists in upward rotation	Small muscle best suited as an intrathoracic flap
Rectus abdominis	Pubis	Costal cartilages of ribs 5–7, xiphoid process of sternum	Superior epigastric artery supply and the deep inferior epigastric artery	Segmentally by thoracoabdominal nerves (T7–T12)	Flexion of trunk/lumbar vertebrae postural muscle. Assists with breathing. Helps create intra-abdominal pressure	Lower anterior chest wall. Some muscle atrophy occurs owing to denervation. If based on superior epigastric, adequate blood flow by way of the internal mammary artery required
External oblique	Fleshy digitations from lower 8 costae. Broad, thin, and irregularly quadrilateral, its muscular portion occupying the side	Lower iliac crest. Inguinal ligament. Upper aponeurosis anterior abdominal wall, decussates at the linea alba with contralateral fibers	Lower thoracic intercostal vessels	Intercostal nerves T5, T6, T7, T8, T9, T10, T11, subcostal nerve T12	Rotates torso	Upper abdomen and lower thoracic defects as far as the inframammary fold

intercostal spaces are occupied by the intercostal glands in relation to the vessels, unite, form a trunk, and drain in the case of the lower 5 spaces into the cisterna chyli, while upper spaces of the left side end in the thoracic duct and those of the upper right side in the right lymphatic duct.

Sympathetic Nerves

The sympathetic chain courses vertically over the heads of the ribs, just lateral to the radiate

ligaments. The T1 sympathetic ganglion fuses with C7 and C8 to form the stellate ganglion, slightly above the first rib lying transversely and medially.

Chest Wall Movement

The easiest model to express the mechanics of quiet respiration is a cylinder (the sternum, ribs, cartilages, and vertebrae) with the diaphragm piston (see **Fig. 6**). There are 3 inspiratory actions

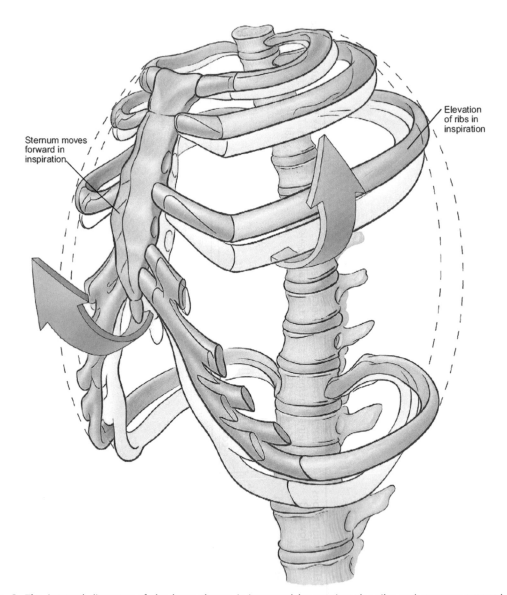

Sternum moves forward in inspiration

Elevation of ribs in inspiration

Fig. 8. The internal diameter of the bony thorax is increased by moving the ribs and sternum upward and outward to increase the inspiratory volume, and is decreased by moving the ribs and sternum downward and inward. Contraction of the accessory muscles of the inspiration increases in thoracic diameter, whereas the accessory muscles of expiration decrease the thoracic volume by moving the ribs and sternum downward and inward. (*From* Graeber GM, Nazim M. The anatomy of the ribs and the sternum and their relationship to chest wall structure and function. Thorac Surg Clin 2007;17(4):473–89; with permission.)

of the diaphragm related to the cranial-caudal orientation of the muscle fibers and the existence of the zone of opposition (the area of contact between the diaphragm and the rib cage). First, as the diaphragm contracts it pulls the central tendon in a caudal direction, thus expanding chest volumes (piston-like action). At the same time it pushes the abdominal organs down and increases the intra-abdominal pressure, which is transmitted across the apposition zone, pushing the lower ribs outward, resulting in expansion of the rib cage. Finally, the relationship of the contracting, descending diaphragm with the opposing effect of the abdominal contents serves as a fulcrum. The net effect is force exerted on the lower ribs cranially, resulting in their upward and outward movement all because of its unique elliptical cylinder capped by a dome shape.[5]

The lungs, which are in direct contact with the chest wall via the pleural surfaces, follow the generated negative extrathoracic pressure and expand. Once inspiration is complete the diaphragm relaxes, and the intrinsic elastic component of the lungs causes them to contract toward their original volume, causing exhalation.

Motion of the skeletal components of the chest wall facilitates the changes in the dimensions of the cylinder (the chest) (**Fig. 8**). The ribs and costal cartilages act as bucket handles that move up and down on the spine. Anteriorly, the ribs are connected to the sternum, which can be viewed as a mechanical pump handle. The joint between the manubrium and the body of the sternum allows the body to have a greater anterior and cephalad excursion, which causes the lower ribs to move more cephalad and anterior than the upper ribs, resulting in a greater increase in diameter in the lower chest.

The volume shifts of the cylinder can be increased greatly during times of need. The accessory muscles of respiration, using the mechanism mentioned earlier, respond to increase the diameter of the chest on inspiration (sternocleidomastoid muscle, the scalene muscles, and the external intercostals). The accessory muscles of expiration (internal intercostal, rectus abdominis, external and internal oblique, and transverse abdominis muscles) function to decrease the internal thoracic diameters and decrease the volume of the cylinder, hence forcing the chest to exhale air. These muscles cause the ribs and the sternum to move downward. The abdominal muscles force the viscera cephalad, pushing the diaphragm upward. These changes, along with increased respiratory rate, allow a tremendous increase in respiratory gas exchange to deal with the increased demand.

Because of their fiber orientations and the distances between their costal insertions and the center of rotation of the ribs, the conventional view is that the external intercostal muscles elevate the ribs and have an inspiratory action, whereas the internal intercostals lower the ribs and so have an expiratory action. This view may not be completely accurate, as animal studies suggest that the position (both craniocaudally and dorsoventrally), lung volume, and interaction with other spaces can affect their action.[6]

The exact contribution and interaction of the thoracic rib cage (principally intercostals), abdominal rib cage (principally diaphragm), and abdominal muscles were historically difficult to study noninvasively and dynamically. But more recently sound data have become available on the interaction and contributions of these compartments at rest and after different forms of exercise.[7] Significant abnormal patterns at rest and after exercise, and asynchronies between compartments have been recognized in disease states.[8] However, the local and global changes after chest wall resection and reconstruction are yet to be studied in such detail. Early evidence from pectus excavatum patients suggest that patterns of disordered chest wall motion are present in subgroups of patients, but whether surgical correction improves this is uncertain.[9]

REFERENCES

1. Gray H. Gray's anatomy: the anatomical basis of medicine and surgery. 39th edition. London: Churchill-Livingston; 2002.
2. Robertson CH, Eschenbacher WL, Johnson RL, et al. Respiratory muscle blood flow distribution during expiratory resistance. J Clin Invest 1977;60:473–80.
3. Rochester DF. The diaphragm: contractile properties and fatigue. J Clin Invest 1985;75(5):1397–402.
4. Miller JI Jr. Muscles of the chest wall. Thorac Surg Clin 2007;17(4):463–72.
5. De Troyer A. The respiratory muscles. In: Crystal RG, editor. The lung: scientific foundation. Philadelphia: Lippincott Raven; 1997. p. 1203–15.
6. De Troyer A, Kirkwood PA, Wilson TA. Respiratory action of the intercostal muscles. Physiol Rev 2005; 85(2):717–56.
7. Aliverti A, Pedotti A. Opto-electronic plethysmography. Monaldi Arch Chest Dis 2003;59(1):12–6.
8. Aliverti A, Quaranta M, Chakrabarti B, et al. Paradoxical movement of the lower ribcage at rest and during exercise in COPD patients. Eur Respir J 2009;33(1): 49–60.
9. Herrmann KA, Zech C, Strauss T, et al. [Cine MRI of the thorax in patients with pectus excavatum]. Radiologe 2006;46(4):309–16 [in German].

Principles of Chest Wall Resection and Reconstruction

Pasquale Ferraro, MD[a],*, Sabrina Cugno, MD[b],
Moishe Liberman, MD CM, PhD[a],
Michel Alain Danino, MD, PhD[b], Patrick G. Harris, MD CM[c]

KEYWORDS

- Chest wall resection • Chest wall reconstruction
- En bloc resection • Functional outcome

Despite significant improvements in surgical technique and perioperative care, the management of patients requiring chest wall resection and reconstruction is an ongoing challenge for thoracic surgeons. Whether the indication be neoplastic or nonneoplastic, in most cases surgery remains the mainstay of therapy and a collaborative approach with reconstructive plastic surgeons is essential in obtaining good results. Malignant tumors of the chest wall represent the greatest challenge, and the modern-day approach to these patients requires multidisciplinary consultation with oncologists dedicated to this specific field.

HISTORICAL NOTE

Pioneering work on chest wall resections primary tumors was first reported by Clagett from the Mayo Clinic in 1957.[1] In wartime, surgeons gained experience in the management of chest wall trauma and flail chest, and developed the general principles of chest wall stabilization. Experience with malignancies involving the chest wall was first obtained from patients with lung cancer or breast cancer with direct invasion of the underlying soft tissues or bony structures, or from patients with metastatic lesions as reported by Martini and colleagues from Memorial Sloan Kettering in New York.[2] Over the years, Pairolero and Arnold, also from the Mayo Clinic, set the standards for surgical resection and reconstruction of the chest wall as well as for oncologic results and long-term functional outcomes.[3–5]

INDICATIONS FOR RESECTION

Indications for chest wall resection and reconstruction are numerous and varied. Resection of the chest wall is most often required as a curative approach to patients presenting with a lesion or tumor of the bony structures or soft tissues. Other indications for resection with curative intent range from congenital disorders, the most common being pectus type malformation, to a variety of infectious and/or inflammatory disorders such as abscesses or osteomyelitis (Table 1). Radionecrosis secondary to locoregional treatment of breast cancer has fortunately seen its incidence decrease significantly over the years with the advent of linear accelerators. Tumors of the chest wall include both benign and malignant lesions, which in turn may be primary or secondary. Direct invasion of the chest wall by lung or breast cancer continue to represent the most common indication for chest wall resection as reported by several investigators.[6,7] Primary tumors of the chest wall, whether their origin be soft tissue or bony/cartilage, generally represent less than 30% of the indications for

[a] Division of Thoracic Surgery, Department of Surgery, Centre Hospitalier de l'Université de Montreal, Université de Montreal, 1560 Sherbrooke Street East, Montreal, Quebec H2L 4M1, Canada
[b] Division of Plastic and Reconstructive Surgery, Department of Surgery, Centre Hospitalier de l'Université de Montreal, Université de Montreal, 1560 Sherbrooke Street East, Montreal, Quebec H2L 4M1, Canada
[c] Department of Surgery, Centre Hospitalier de l'Université de Montreal, Université de Montreal, Montreal, Quebec, Canada
* Corresponding author.
E-mail address: pasquale.ferraro@umontreal.ca

Thorac Surg Clin 20 (2010) 465–473
doi:10.1016/j.thorsurg.2010.07.008
1547-4127/10/$ — see front matter © 2010 Elsevier Inc. All rights reserved.

Table 1
Indications for chest wall resection
Congenital Disorders
Pectus excavatum
Pectus carinatum
Poland syndrome
Sternal defects
Infectious/Inflammatory
Osteomyelitis
Tuberculosis
Actinomycosis
Blastomycosis
Radionecrosis
Trauma
Neoplastic lesions
Benign
Malignant
Primary
Direct invasion (lung, breast, mediastinum, skin)
Secondary/metastatic

resection. A histologic classification of the most common primary tumors is presented in **Table 2**.

In certain rare circumstances, chest wall resection may be indicated for palliative control of an infected or ulcerated cancer or for pain management in a patient who is otherwise inoperable. Resection may also be required for metastatic disease; its exact role, however, remains

Table 2	
Classification of primary chest wall tumors	
Benign Primary Tumors	**Malignant Primary Tumors**
Bone and cartilage:	Bone and cartilage:
Osteochondroma	Chondrosarcoma
Chondroma	Osteosarcoma
Enchondroma	Ewing sarcoma
Fibrous dysplasia	Plasmacytoma
Eosinophilic	Lymphoma
granuloma	Askin tumor (PNET)
Granular cell tumor	Soft tissue:
Chondroblastoma	Malignant fibrous
Soft tissue:	histiocytoma
Lipoma	Leiomyosarcoma
Fibroma	Liposarcoma
Neurofibroma	Fibrosarcoma
Lymphangioma	Desmoid tumor
Hemangioma	Rhabdomyosarcoma
	Neurofibrosarcoma

controversial and in many cases surgery is either solely diagnostic or palliative in nature.

CLINICAL FEATURES AND INVESTIGATION

Proper and complete patient workup is required before undertaking any chest wall resection. A careful history-taking and physical examination will look for prior malignancy, radiation therapy, recent trauma, or hereditary conditions (eg, Gardner syndrome, Von Recklinghausen disease). It is also important to note the presence of pain and systemic signs such as fever, diaphoresis, or weight loss as well as the pattern of growth if a palpable mass is present. As reported by Burt,[8] pain with or without a mass is present in more than 50% of patients with primary bony or cartilaginous tumors. On physical examination, key features include size and location of the lesion, surrounding and underlying structures, and the presence or absence of locoregional lymph nodes.

Radiographic workup of patients presenting with lesions of the chest wall has evolved significantly over recent years from plain radiographs and nuclear medicine bone scans. The combined use of computed tomography (CT), magnetic resonance imaging (MRI), and positron emission tomography (PET) scans helps establish in most patients the type of the lesion, neoplastic versus nonneoplastic, as well as the nature of the tumor, benign versus malignant, if a tumor is present.[9–12] CT scan of the chest is useful in establishing the exact size, characteristics, and location of a lesion, while MRI generally provides more accurate imaging of tumor extent, invasion of blood vessels or brachial plexus, and involvement of the spinal cord. PET scanning has proved useful in establishing the nature of the primary lesion as well as for looking for distant metastases. These imaging modalities are also useful in guiding physicians with proper patient management regarding medical versus surgical therapy. These methods, however, have not obviated the need to accurately confirm tissue diagnosis with some form of biopsy in the great majority of patients.

Finally, in the presence of a primary chest wall tumor in an elderly patient, the workup must address the issue of surgical candidacy. Appropriate testing may be required to establish cardiopulmonary reserve and to rule out important underlying disease such as coronary artery disease or severe emphysema.

DIAGNOSIS AND BIOPSY

The importance of obtaining an accurate preoperative tissue diagnosis cannot be overstated. In certain circumstances, the lesion may be benign and not require resection, making a surgical approach necessary only for diagnosis. In other cases, the lesion may be best treated with a nonsurgical approach even if it is found to be a malignant tumor (so-called medical tumor), as is the case with solitary plasmacytoma, Ewing sarcoma, lymphoma, or metastatic disease.[13–15]

Preoperative diagnosis is also essential in patients requiring an extensive resection and complex reconstruction. The ulcerated and infected lesion shown in **Fig. 1** was confirmed on biopsy in the authors' institution to be a recurrent high-grade fibrosarcoma. The successful resection of this tumor and reconstruction of the spine and chest wall was possible only through the careful planning and collaboration of the neurosurgical, plastic, and thoracic surgery teams. Over the last decade, the use of neoadjuvant therapy in the management of chest wall tumors has become more common as reported by Walsh and colleagues from M.D. Anderson.[16] Neoadjuvant therapy may be indicated in certain tumors located in areas where the proximity of vital structures limits the extent of the resection, as shown in **Fig. 2**, in large bulky tumors, or in high-grade sarcomas with poor short-term prognosis. In this setting tissue diagnosis is systematically required.

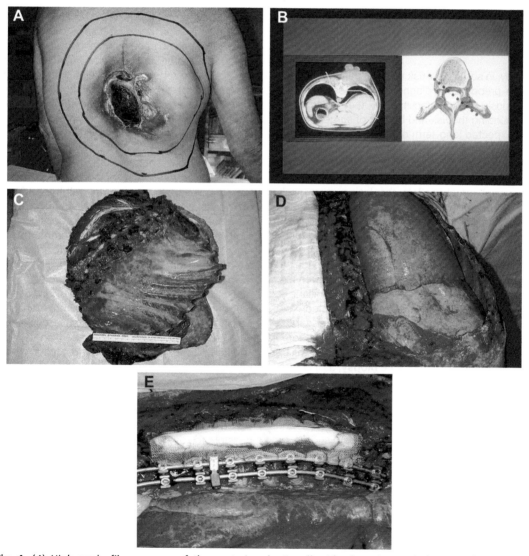

Fig. 1. (*A*) High-grade fibrosarcoma of the posterior chest wall with ulceration and chronic infection. Skin drawing depicting the extent of the tumor and the resection margins. (*B*) Intended resection including vertebral body. (*C*) Surgical specimen. (*D*) Defect in chest wall showing underlying structures. (*E*) Spine stabilization and reconstruction.

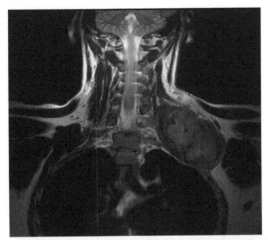

Fig. 2. MR image of a desmoid tumor involving the left supraclavicular space, left neck, and shoulder area in proximity to the brachial plexus.

Finally, in some high-risk surgical patients, obtaining a preoperative diagnosis helps establish the prognosis and facilitates the discussion surrounding the risk and benefit of surgery versus the expected long-term outcome for the patient.

When deciding on what type of biopsy to perform, it is necessary to first consider several factors. How large is the lesion and is it located near vital structures? Is the lesion more likely benign or malignant, and if malignant is surgery with curative intent an option? Is neoadjuvant therapy being considered? Is the patient elderly and at high risk for an extensive chest wall resection? Once the decision has been made to proceed with a biopsy, the surgeon must ensure that sufficient tissue is obtained, that spillage is avoided, that tissue planes are respected, and that the biopsy incision is well located for subsequent removal at the time of definitive resection.

In most cases, the first biopsy attempted will be a **fine-needle or core needle biopsy,** as it is safe, easily performed on an outpatient basis, nontraumatic, and associated with minimal spillage. In experienced hands, the diagnostic accuracy has been reported as high as 92% by Welker and colleagues.[17] An **excisional biopsy** should be considered when a needle biopsy is nondiagnostic, when the lesion is well situated and less than 5 cm in diameter, when the lesion is probably benign, or when the lesion is nonsurgical (metastasis, medical tumor, palliative intent). In such cases, a 1- to 2-cm margin is sufficient with primary closure using local surrounding tissue. The patient may subsequently require reoperation for wide radical resection if the lesion is proved to be a primary malignant tumor. An **incisional biopsy** is required for tumors larger than 5 cm,

for tumors located in a difficult area such as the axilla or supraclavicular space, or for patients requiring neoadjuvant therapy, again in the setting of a nondiagnostic needle biopsy.

SURGICAL RESECTION

Surgical resection of a primary malignant tumor of the chest wall requires careful planning and execution, as most patients only get one chance for cure and reoperation for recurrent tumor or for a failed operation is generally associated with poor outcomes. When surgery is curative, the resection must be a wide en bloc radical excision of the tumor with adequate margins. The extent of the resection should not be limited by the size of the resulting defect. The en bloc resection includes the skin and soft tissue overlying the tumor, involved rib or sternum, and any underlying, attached structure such as lung, pericardium, or diaphragm. In rare cases, invasion of the liver by a sarcoma of the chest wall has been documented.[18] In an example from the authors' institution shown in **Fig. 3**, the patient with a high-grade chondrosarcoma underwent a wide radical en bloc resection of the chest wall and diaphragm, and an extended right hepatectomy with negative margins. The patient, who did not receive any form of adjuvant therapy, is well with no evidence of disease at 10-year follow-up. When planning the resection of ribs, it is important to consider that tumor spread is possible through the marrow or along the periosteum of an involved rib. In general a 4- to 5-cm margin, as shown in **Fig. 4**, is recommended for primary malignant tumors.[4,8,19] For metastatic tumors or for palliative resections, a 2-cm margin is usually sufficient. Obtaining negative margins on frozen section is necessary in all cases to ensure complete resection.

When performing a chest wall resection for an infectious or inflammatory process, the same basic principles apply. Margins must be wide enough to obtain healthy viable tissue at the borders of the wound to ensure proper healing. In some cases of deeply situated lesions it may be possible to save the overlying intact skin to facilitate closure.

PRINCIPLES OF CHEST WALL RECONSTRUCTION
Introduction

While the inception of chest wall reconstruction can be traced to Tansini's descriptive report on the use of a pedicled latissimus dorsi for coverage of an anterior thoracic defect,[20] coverage of chest wall defects has since evolved to include the full

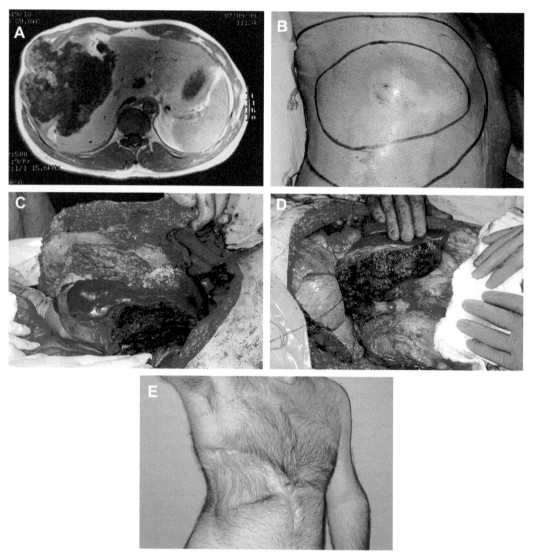

Fig. 3. (*A*) MR image of chest wall tumor invading the liver. (*B*) Skin drawing depicting the extent of the tumor and intended resection. (*C*) Operative field showing tumor invasion of the liver. (*D*) Operative field once the resection has been completed. (*E*) Final result following chest wall and abdominal wall reconstruction 2 years after surgery.

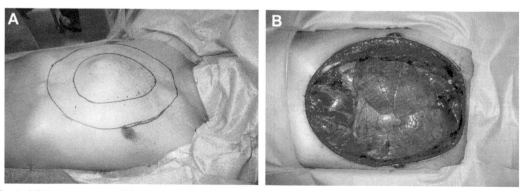

Fig. 4. (*A*) Osteosarcoma of the sternum shown with depiction of resection margins. (*B*) Operative field following radical en bloc sternectomy with resection of the clavicles, pericardium, and diaphragm.

range of tissue transfer in the armamentarium of the reconstructive surgeon. The goals of chest wall reconstruction are twofold. While priority is given to the restoration of functional and structural integrity, the ultimate aesthetics of the reconstruction is likewise an integral component of the end result. Consequent of extensive extirpation of chest wall tumors, the resultant deficit may lead to loss of rigid support requisite to inspiratory function, as well as visceral protection. An algorithmic approach to chest wall reconstruction begins with the assessment of the nature of the defect, taking into consideration factors such as infection, tumor extirpation, previous radiation therapy, and surgical intervention. The latter factors bear influence on the type of tissue required, as well as whether reconstruction can be performed in a single stage or whether it is better delayed pending eradication of conflicting factors. Second, the location and depth of the defect is considered, as anterolateral defects have a bearing on respiratory mechanics, often requiring alloplastic material to reestablish structural support. Furthermore, defect location dictates regional flap use. For the given regional flaps available, aesthetic considerations as well as donor site morbidity are evaluated. Finally, patient factors, including lifestyle and work as well as prognosis, are considered to determine the best reconstructive option (**Table 3**).

Restoration of Skeletal Support

Following a detailed assessment of the defect and assessment of the patient's ventilatory status, successful reconstruction mandates reestablishment of skeletal integrity and a well-vascularized composite reconstruction, which provides both exterior coverage and fill of any existent dead space. Although the former is dependent on the patient's baseline functional capacity, classic doctrine states that a deficiency of 2 ribs can be compensated by adequate soft tissue reconstruction; however, loss of more than 4 consecutive ribs or defects of the lateral chest wall larger than 5 cm necessitate skeletal stabilization to avert a flail-chest deformity.[21] Options for skeletal reconstruction include either autogenous or alloplastic reconstruction. The convenience, reliability, and ease of application of synthetic materials have relegated the use of autologous materials for structural repair chiefly to the realm of historical significance. Alloplastic materials include Vicryl, Prolene, or Marlex mesh, polytetrafluoroethylene (Gore-Tex), as well as a composite of mesh and methyl methacrylate (**Fig. 5**).[5,22] Moreover, AlloDerm, an acellular human cadaveric dermal matrix, has proved promising as an alternative structural buttress.

Soft Tissue Reconstruction

For chest wall soft tissue coverage, skin grafts or local random or axial fasciocutaneous flaps (eg, thoracoepigastric flap) have a limited role. Thus, priority is given to locally available options provided by muscle or musculocutaneous flaps. The latter include the latissimus dorsi, pectoralis major, rectus abdominis, serratus anterior, and external oblique. In the rare circumstance where no tissue is available locally free tissue transfer can be considered, which includes either contralateral chest wall or lower limb fasciocutaneous or muscle-musculocutaneous flaps.[23] Microsurgical tissue transfer has been facilitated by the use of interposition vein grafts to effectively bridge the gap between recipient and donor vessels, thereby eliminating pedicle length as an impediment to flap selection. The selection of the appropriate tissue transfer necessitates evaluation of surgical scars, which may provide valuable information regarding prior ablation of regional flaps or their vascular pedicles, the location of the

Table 3
Factors to consider for chest wall reconstruction
Size and location of defect
Depth of defect
Quality of surrounding tissues
Infection
Radionecrosis
Residual tumor
Patient lifestyle and work
Prognosis and long-term survival
Palliative resection

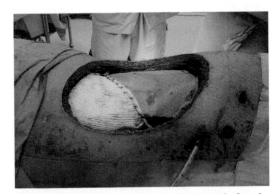

Fig. 5. Reconstruction with a Prolene mesh for the chest wall and a Gore-Tex mesh for the diaphragm and abdominal wall.

defect, need for prosthetic material or viscera coverage, and whether additional tissue bulk is required to fill a dead space void.[24]

Among the aforementioned muscle and musculocutaneous flaps, the latissimus dorsi is considered the workhorse in chest wall reconstruction, as this flap enables coverage of the entire ipsilateral chest wall.[25] Recent improvement in surgical technique now allows the latissimus dorsi to be harvested with the patient in a supine position, which avoids unnecessary changes in positioning. Moreover, flap survival based on collateral retrograde flow through the serratus branch presents a considerable advantage, as previous trauma to the dominant pedicle, the thoracodorsal artery, does not obviate use of this flap. Of note, the subscapular trunk, from which the thoracodorsal artery derives, enables concomitant harvest of the latissimus dorsi muscle, along with serratus anterior, and a skin island based on the circumflex scapular vessels. The latter chimeric flap design permits reconstruction of complex defects for which tissue demand is greater.

The pectoralis major is considered the principal flap for sternal and anterosuperior chest wall defect coverage.[26–28] The vascularization to this flap is either through its dominant thoracoacromial pedicle, or based on the first through sixth intercostal perforating branches arising from the internal mammary artery. This dual vascular pattern permits the use of only the medial two-thirds of muscle, thereby sparing the lateral third and anterior axillary fold. Moreover, complete release of the pectoralis major muscle from its bony connections permits mobilization as an island flap based on the thoracoacromial pedicle, extending the reach of this flap to the xiphoid process, thereby obliterating the entire anterior mediastinal space.[29]

The rectus abdominis flap, based on either the deep superior or inferior epigastric system, affords unparalleled versatility of skin island design (ie, vertically transversely oriented skin paddle), which has enabled wide application of this flap for coverage of anterior or anterolateral defects. While perforator flaps of the anterior abdominal wall have gained popularity for breast reconstruction, in view of the recognized donor site morbidity following rectus abdominis muscle harvest, similar enthusiasm for chest wall reconstruction has been tempered by the less reliable vascularity and consequences of resultant flap failure. The latter flaps are considered the principal tissue transfers for chest wall reconstruction. In addition, the external oblique myocutaneous flap has a role for coverage of lower anterior chest wall defects, based on segmental blood supply from the lateral

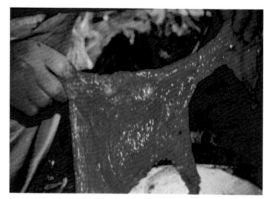

Fig. 6. Greater omentum pedicled flap.

cutaneous branches of the inferior 8 posterior intercostal arteries.

The greater omentum maintains a chief role in chest wall reconstruction (**Fig. 6**).[26,30,31] This pedicled flap may be based on either right or left gastroepiploic arteries, and pedicle lengthening by its release from the transverse colon and stomach allows transposition of this flap to virtually any chest wall location. Although its versatility has been widely appreciated, flap harvest presents significant potential intra-abdominal morbidity; further, the friable nature of omental tissue may render flap inset difficult. Moreover, it is difficult to accurately predict flap size preoperatively because no direct correlation exists between the volume of the greater omentum and the morphologic characteristics of the patient.[32]

Pleural Cavity Management

Although discussion has focused on skeletal support and soft tissue coverage, management of the pleural cavity, to obliterate postpneumonectomy empyema spaces, and for closure of bronchopleural or tracheoesophageal fistulas, for instance, is often essential. Omentum, as well as locally available muscle flaps including pectoralis major, rectus abdominis, latissimus dorsi, and serratus, have been described for such purposes and can be placed within the intrathoracic cavity through 4- to 5-cm defects with a 2-rib resection.[33] In addition to the omentum, the rhomboid major has been noted as a valuable alternative for intrathoracic cavity obliteration if previous thoracotomy precludes the use of regional muscle flaps.[24]

SUMMARY

When dealing with lesions or tumors of the chest wall requiring a complex resection and reconstruction, a multidisciplinary approach offers the greatest chance for success. This approach includes a thorough assessment of the patient and the lesion, an adequate biopsy to confirm tissue diagnosis, and a well-established treatment plan. In the case of a primary tumor of the chest wall, the extent of the resection should not be limited by the size of the resulting defect. Following resection, chest wall reconstruction mandates an appreciation for restoration of functional and structural components. The nature of the defect must be carefully assessed, and several factors such as infection and previous radiation therapy must be considered. These factors bear influence on the type of tissue required as well as whether reconstruction can be performed in a single stage or as a 2-staged procedure. Finally, aesthetic considerations, donor site morbidity, and patient factors, including lifestyle and work as well as prognosis, are considered to determine the best reconstructive option.

More detailed reviews of the surgical management of neoplastic and nonneoplastic lesions of the chest wall as well as specific techniques of chest wall reconstruction are presented elsewhere in this issue and thus are not covered extensively in this article.

REFERENCES

1. Pascuzzi CA, Dahlia DC, Clagget OT. Primary tumors of the ribs and sternum. Surg Gynecol Obstet 1957;104:390.
2. Martini N, McCormack PM, Bains MS. Chest wall tumors: clinical results of treatment. Major challenges. In: Grillo HC, Eschapasse H, editors. International trends in general thoracic surgery, vol. 2. Philadelphia: Saunders; 1987. p. 285.
3. Pairolero PC, Arnold PG. Chest wall tumors: experience with 100 consecutive patients. J Thorac Cardiovasc Surg 1985;90:367.
4. King RM, Pairolero PC, Trastek VF, et al. Primary chest wall tumors: factors affecting survival. Ann Thorac Surg 1986;41:597.
5. Arnold PG, Pairolero PC. Chest wall reconstruction: an account of 500 consecutive patients. Plast Reconstr Surg 1996;98:804.
6. Mansour KA, Thourani VH, Losken A, et al. Chest wall resections and reconstruction: a 25-year experience. Ann Thorac Surg 2002;73:1720.
7. Weyant MJ, Bains MS, Venkatraman E, et al. Results of chest wall resection and reconstruction with and without rigid prosthesis. Ann Thorac Surg 2006;81: 279.
8. Burt M. Primary malignant tumors of the chest wall. Chest Surg Clin N Am 1994;4:137.
9. Fortier M, Mayo JR, Swensen SJ, et al. MR imaging of chest wall lesions. Radiographics 1994;1:597.
10. Dillman JR, Pernicano PG, McHugh JB, et al. Cross-sectional imaging of primary thoracic sarcomas with histopathologic correlation: a review for the radiologist. Curr Probl Diagn Radiol 2010;39(1):17.
11. Shin DS, Shon OJ, Han DS, et al. The clinical efficacy of (18)F-FDG-PET/CT in benign and malignant musculoskeletal tumours. Ann Nucl Med 2008;22(7): 603.
12. Tian R, Su M, Tian Y, et al. Dual-time point PET/CT with F-18 FDG for the differentiation of malignant and benign bone lesions. Skeletal Radiol 2009; 38(5):451.
13. Shamberger RC, Laquaglia MP, Krailo MD, et al. Ewing sarcoma of the rib: results of an intergroup study with analysis of outcome by timing of resection. J Thorac Cardiovasc Surg 2000;119:1154.
14. Holland J, Trenkner DA, Wasserman TH, et al. Plasmacytoma: treatment results and conversion to myeloma. Cancer 1992;69:1513.
15. Dimopoulos MA, Goldstein J, Fuller L, et al. Curability of solitary bone plasmacytoma. J Clin Oncol 1992;10:587.
16. Walsh GL, Davis BM, Swisher SG, et al. A single-institutional, multidisciplinary approach to primary sarcomas involving the chest wall requiring full-thickness resections. J Thorac Cardiovasc Surg 2001;121:48.
17. Welker JA, Henshaw RM, Jelinek J, et al. The percutaneous needle biopsy is safe and recommended in the diagnosis of musculoskeletal masses. Cancer 2000;89:2677.
18. Noiseux N, Ferraro P, Busque S, et al. Chest wall and liver resection for chondrosarcoma. Ann Thorac Surg 2002;74(2):598.
19. McAfee MK, Pairolero PC, Bergstralh EJ, et al. Chondrosarcoma of the chest wall: factors affecting survival. Ann Thorac Surg 1985;40:535.
20. Tansini I. Sopra il mio processo di amputazione della mammella. Gazz Med Ital Torino 1906;57:141 [in Italian].
21. Din AM, Evans GR. Chest wall reconstruction. In: McCarthy JB, Galiano RD, Boutros S, editors. Current therapy in plastic surgery. Philadelphia: Saunders; 2006. p. 362.
22. Deschamps C, Timaksiz BM, Darbandi R, et al. Early and long term results of prosthetic chest wall reconstruction. J Thorac Cardiovasc Surg 1999;117:588.
23. Cordeiro PG, Santamaria E, Hidalgo D. The role of microsurgery in reconstruction of oncologic chest wall defects. Plast Reconstr Surg 2001;108:1924.
24. Netscher DT, Baumholtz MA. Chest reconstruction: I. Anterior and anterolateral chest wall and wounds affecting respiratory function. Plast Reconstr Surg 2009;124:240.
25. Bostwick J, Nahai F, Wallace JG, et al. Sixty latissimus dorsi flaps. Plast Reconstr Surg 1979;63:31.

26. Arnold PG, Pairolero PC. Use of pectoralis muscle flaps to repair defects of the anterior chest wall. Plast Reconstr Surg 1979;63:205.

27. Jones G, Jurkiewicz MJ, Bostwick J, et al. Management of the infected median sternotomy wound with muscle flaps. The Emory 20-year experience. Ann Surg 1997;225:766.

28. Nahai F, Morales L Jr, Bone DK, et al. Pectoralis major muscle turnover flaps for closure of the infected sternotomy wound with preservation of form and function. Plast Reconstr Surg 1982;70:471.

29. Brutus JP, Nikolis A, Perrault I, et al. The unilateral pectoralis major island flap, an efficient and straightforward procedure for reconstruction of full-length sternal defects after post-operative mediastinal wound infection. Br J Plast Surg 2004;56:803.

30. Jurkiewicz MJ, Arnold PG. The omentum: an account of its use in reconstruction of the chest wall. Ann Surg 1977;185:548.

31. Hultman CS, Culbertson JH, Jones GE, et al. Thoracic reconstruction with the omentum: indications, complications and results. Ann Plast Surg 2001;46:242.

32. Skoracki RJ, Chang DW. Reconstruction of the chest wall and thorax. J Surg Oncol 2006;94:455.

33. Losken A, Thourani VH, Carlson GW, et al. A reconstructive algorithm for plastic surgery following extensive chest wall resection. Br J Plast Surg 2004;54:295.

Surgical Management of Chest Wall Trauma

Tamas F. Molnar, MD, PhD

KEYWORDS

- Penetrating chest trauma • Blunt chest trauma
- Flail chest • Chest wound • Blast injuries
- Damage control in thoracic surgery

"...He looks at me wanly.
  The bandages are brown,
  Brown with mud, red only—
  But how deep a red! in the breast of the shirt,
  Deepening red too, as each whistling breath
   Is drawn with the suck of a slow-filling squirt
   While waxen cheeks waste to the pallor of death..."

                    Robert Nichols: Casualty (1916)[1]

The title of this article emphasizes a major factor in the management of thoracic trauma since nonsurgical treatment of thoracic trauma is as much an integral part of the management of chest wall trauma as it is the surgical treatment. Accordingly, the old motto—"A good surgeon knows how to operate; a great surgeon knows when to operate. The best surgeon knows when not to operate"— still holds true. In fact, the treatment of acute conditions of the osteomuscular components of the thoracic cage is shared among thoracic surgeons and trauma and orthopedic specialists, while, in a significant number of severely injured patients, the intensivist and the pulmonologist have the final word.[2] Thoracic trauma comprises 10% to 15% of all traumas, and 30% to 55% percent of polytraumas involve the chest wall. Reportedly, 10% to 15% of blunt chest trauma will result in a flail chest, with an overall mortality around 20%.[3,4] The United Kingdom represents rather a typical example than an exception, where about some 5% of polytrauma patients with associated chest injury are treated primarily by thoracic surgeons.[5]

BASIC ANATOMICOCLINICAL CONSIDERATIONS

The bony thorax is protected by thick layers of muscles at the back of the body and the shoulders. Therefore, the chest wall is more vulnerable laterally and anteriorly, where the intercostal muscles and underlying structure—made of a thin layer of fat, connective tissue and parietal pleura—are left relatively uncovered by voluminous external muscles.[6] The musculo-tendineo-chondral-bony complex of the thoracic wall provides a triple defense against injuries. It has the flexibility of a suspension cable or chain bridge while preserving the rigidity of the body and cemented pillars.[7] The muscles serve as the suspending chain of a drawbridge, adjusting the main rigid body of the bridge against the different forces to which it is exposed. The ribs, built on the vertebral column, are connecting and fixing the body of sternum, like the metal rings of a barrel. The shoulder girdle, clavicle, and scapula are joined to the sternum by semirigid symphysis. Caudally, the entire system is open to the abdominal cavity, being separated only by the diaphragm. If needed, the intercostal muscles and scalenus muscles provide a further reserve for volume—force adjustment. Consequently, the whole complex has a potential to compensate excessive forces, while it lacks the disadvantages of the nonadjustable volume of similar shell-like protective structures like the skull.

Nowadays, extensive chest wall injury, usually in combination with concomitant intrathoracic organ trauma, is gaining more attention because of the changing face of major trauma profiles.[8] Terror

The author has no conflicts of interest to disclose.
Thoracic Surgical Unit, Department of Surgery, University of Pécs, Ifjusag u 13 Pécs, Hungary
E-mail address: tfmolnar@gmail.com

Thorac Surg Clin 20 (2010) 475–485
doi:10.1016/j.thorsurg.2010.07.004

attacks on civilians and novel explosive techniques in modern asymmetric warfare are both responsible for an increased proportion of complex chest wall injuries.[9] A destroyed thoracic wall is a manual book case for damage control,[10] whereby surgical aggressivity should be optimized to ensure restoration and securing of vital functions instead of an immediate and complete regaining of all functions and anatomical integrity.[11] Both civilian practice and military practice are limited by available resources, suffering from a sort of disequilibrium between workload and manpower. In fact, while the military environment is characterized by the unpredictable number of cases and timing of the tide of injured patients (intake), in the civilian practice there is often a scarcity of thoracic surgeons. During management of major trauma, the chest wall loses importance as a protective shell, since the artificial ventilation makes physiological pleural pressure difference irrelevant. Profuse bleeding, however, represents the only acute situation when an immediate surgical approach is often necessary to restore hemodynamic stability and avoid the creation of a clotted hemothorax, which may get infected and generate sepsis at a later date.[12]

CLINICAL CORRELATES

In spite of the common nature of chest injuries (up to 15% of all trauma admissions), most do not require any surgical intervention.[4] In fact, out of 4205 patients with chest trauma from Turkey, only 252 (6%) required a thoracotomy.[2]

It is customary to categorize thoracic injuries into nonpenetrating (blunt) and penetrating (open) ones.[13,14] Nonpenetrating injuries to the chest wall are caused by blunt objects[13,15] or by blast overpressure.[16]

Blunt trauma results from significant compression of the thorax, yielding rib fractures, soft tissue injuries, and intrathoracic damage of different degree due to a stretch-and-shear strain effect. The severity of chest wall injury depends upon the magnitude of compression exerted on the thoracic cage, which, in turn, is closely related to the force and the speed at which the compression occurs. In addition, the direction of blunt chest wall injury is another determining factor of the type of chest wall injury. Blunt traumas impacting the chest wall according to an anteroposterior direction implicate a higher risk of mediastinal injury (aorta, thoracic outlet structures, tracheobronchial, and cardiac), while lateral forces are more likely to generate pleuropulmonary injuries. In order to control severe tracheobronchial bleeding associated with blunt trauma, Nishiumi and

colleagues[17] recently proposed the immediate exclusion of the bronchus by inserting a bronchial blocker. The criteria and the timing for emergency thoracotomy for bleeding remain unclear and may vary depending on the nature of the trauma (ie, penetrating versus blunt injury).[18] The Advanced Trauma Life Support (ATLAS) recommendations for emergency thoracotomy include blood loss of 1500 mL immediately after insertion of the chest tube, continuing blood loss of 200 mL/h for 2 to 4 hours through the chest tube, and resistance to transfused blood.[19] In the event of parenchymal laceration, a lower threshold for preparing for emergency thoracotomy has been suggested (ie, 500 mL in the chest tube), based on the estimation of the anticipated intrathoracic blood loss to be double the amount of blood visible in the collecting unit.[18] Indeed, a dichotomic approach towards bleeding causing blunt compared with penetrating injuries has been proposed. Following blunt trauma, delaying the surgical exploration when the total blood loss is greater than 1000 mL may entail a significant risk for mortality.[20]

Crushing chest wall injuries,[21] most commonly occurring after road traffic accidents, frequently result in multiple rib fractures and flail chest. Compression forces, like blasts[22] or falls and direct blows, can cause similar injuries. Blast injuries, caused by pressure waves, can cause either blunt or open injuries.[23] Although shock waves transmitted by air are mostly absorbed by the thoracic wall, they may cause parenchymal injuries (ie, pneumothorax), while projectiles driven by explosion can induce a penetrating trauma. An acute thoracic compression syndrome (traumatic asphyxia), also known as Olivier syndrome or Perthes syndrome,[24] may ensue when the acting force is greater than 20 G and generates acute venous hypertension with a fatality rate of 40% to 50%. Interestingly, extra loud music, mimicking a blast to the chest wall thereby transmitted to the lung, can represent a possible cause for spontaneous pneumothorax.[25] Not surprisingly, this hypothesis has received immediate attention; however, rupture of the visceral pleura and accumulation of sufficient air in the pleural space, inducing collapse of only one lung, are highly unlikely, as even a sonic bomb (150–170 decibels, 1–3 kPa) does not yield adverse effects on respiratory system.

Open chest wall injuries are usually penetrating thoracic wounds. The chest wall becomes only the first section of a tunnel before the object enters the pleural space and damages inner organs.[2,4,26] While stab wounds are sharp edged cut injuries, shot wounds are caused by different projectiles capable of destroying tissues in irregular cross and horizontal planes due to the combined effect of direct pressure and shock wave, according on their energy and profile parameters.[8] A basic distinction between low-energy and high-energy projectile impacts should be made. Moreover, according to profile characteristics, they can be distinguished in sharp-pointed (ie, bullet-like or nail-shaped) or irregularly shaped objects (ie, shrapnel or splinter). Entry and exit sites are examined carefully to identify with trajectories related to specific tissue damage patterns. Moreover, the effect of the shock waves in the vicinity of the projectile tunnel determines the depth and width of the ensuing necrosis and becomes a major outcome predictor. Of particular concern are foreign bodies brought in or generated by hostile impact. In suicide bomb attacks,[9] bone fragments, either from the victim or from other participants (even the perpetrator's), or pieces of clothing and secondary splinters (ie, car pieces, stones, and debris) represent dangerous hotbeds for secondary inflammation.

DIFFERENT TYPES OF CHEST WALL TRAUMA
Soft Tissue Injuries

Superficial wounds
Blunt trauma may cause skin abrasions, ecchymoses, and hematomas deep in the chest wall layers (**Table 1**).[16,27] Penetrating and tangential injuries may induce punctures and lacerations of trivial significance if the force of chest wall injury is small. From the forensic point of view, it is important to give not only an exact description of the lesion, but also to perform a full excision of the entrance wound and to treat it as a specimen.[28] In this setting, external wounds are misleading, because they may look deceptively innocuous. Hence, these injuries should be explored to their

deepest point to exclude any penetration through the thoracic wall, especially taking into consideration the fact that thoracic wall muscles tend to close spontaneously above a narrow channel or tunnel of injury.

Also, it is important to ascertain the length and width of the cold weapon used. Most stab wounds occur in the left side as they are brought about by a right handed attacker.[29] Posterior stab wounds are less likely to penetrate the chest wall because of the intervening muscle mass. Conversely, stab wounds in the axillary region are more likely to enter the pleural space and proceed further. Knife stabs regularly have straight edges, but also have to be cleaned, debrided and closed if less than six hours old.

Bullet wounds are to be excised and projectiles removed if possible. The latter are highly unlikely to stop in the chest wall: if they do, they are harmless. The surgical attitude is defined not by what has happened to the thoracic wall but by the possible involvement of intrathoracic structures. Through-and-through chest wounds are benign and respond to chest drain and suction treatment in all but the ones falling into proximity of the pulmonary hila, heart, and great vessels.[4,11,14,27]

Extensive chest wall injuries
Significant loss of substance resulting from full-thickness chest wall trauma poses an immediate threat to life only if the source of profuse bleeding is not controlled. Otherwise, cardiopulmonary function can be preserved by artificial ventilation. Sucking chest wounds lead to mediastinal compression, causing distortion of the heart and great vessels. Therefore, a cover the hole and drain the cavity policy as the basic tenet should be followed in such cases.[14,30] The depth, extension, and time scale of soft tissue necrosis and superinfection will determine the final outcome. In this context, a staged, definitive treatment of extensive soft tissue chest wall defects is to be recommended, since there is no need to rush approximating tissues characterized by questionable viability.[11] An immediate and proper debridement should be followed by definite reconstruction when active inflammation is under control and tissue demarcation is complete. Plastic surgical reconstructive principles are to be applied[31] as outlined by other contributors of this issue of *Thoracic Surgery Clinics*.

There are no convincing data about the ideal antibiotic coverage.[32] The available evidence, however, support the use of prophylactic antibiotics to reduce post-traumatic thoracic empyema. In addition, because soft tissue injuries can be more painful than those elicited by fractures of

Table 1
Chest wall injury: relation between anatomy and consequence of injury mechanism

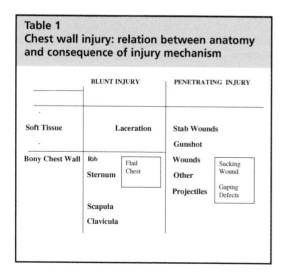

	BLUNT INJURY		PENETRATING INJURY	
Soft Tissue	Laceration		Stab Wounds	
			Gunshot	
Bony Chest Wall	Rib	Flail Chest	Wounds	Sucking Wound
	Sternum		Other	
			Projectiles	Gaping Defects
	Scapula			
	Clavicula			

the bony cage, individualized and effective pain relief protocols need to be devised to avoid hypoventilation-related morbidity.[33]

Surgical emphysema

Surgical or subcutaneous emphysema is usually a sign of a communication between the pleural space or the underlying lung or other hollow organs, such as the tracheobronchial tree and esophagus. In patients with advanced chronic obstructive pulmonary disease (COPD), only a minor trauma is necessary to produce rupture of a bulla with the attendant pneumothorax. The presence of adhesions from previous tuberculosis, pneumonias, or post-traumatic hemothorax may prevent lung collapse and generate a direct communication between the pleural space and the chest wall. Air can be tracked along the bronchial or vascular sheaths and appear as subcutaneous emphysema external to the bony chest cage without causing collapse of the lung. The appearance of mediastinal emphysema extending to the chest wall and the neck following a negligible trauma of minor entity among otherwise young and healthy patients has been reported.[34]

Chest wall superficial crepitations also can be attributed to anaerobic infections[35] caused by a subcutaneous spread originating from minuscule superficial scratches. Anergic patients are a danger for showing no alarming signs of inflammation or severe infection.

If serious underlying causes of surgical emphysema are excluded, a watch-and-wait attitude is advisable. Subcutaneously inserted large bore needles or small-caliber tubes might relieve the harmless tension within the layers of the chest wall and the not so innocent tension of the patients and relatives if due explanation and assurances fail.

Spontaneous haemothorax[36] may originate from tear of intercostal vessels or internal mammary artery as a result of unrecognized blunt chest wall injury. In an era of a nearly pandemic anticoagulation, patients or those who have minor coagulopathy (ie, liver failure due to substance abuse) are prone to develop hemothorax after negligible or undetected injuries.

Impalement

The jury is still out about where and when to remove an indwelling foreign body from the chest wall. Patients are transferred for long distances over a significant time with strange foreign bodies protruding from their thorax. At times, bony segments from the same patient can be dislodged inward to create complex injuries. Present principles of management[19,37] derive from abdominal parenchymal surgery and from experience with injured vessels of extremities. Paramedic handbooks and army field manuals properly warn against the removal of these terrible weapons on the spot. In fact, perforating and embedded foreign bodies might completely fill up the trajectory channel, thereby compressing the surrounding parenchymal and preventing profuse hemorrhage. However, heart and lungs on the other hand do inevitably rub and cut themselves against the sharp edges of indwelling objects during their perpetual movements. Nevertheless, the current prehospitalization protocol, leaving the impaling objects in place, is the only presently accepted method.[37] Preliminary extraction of knives, pointed rods, and similar objects from the chest, followed by insertion of a chest drain of the same size either in their tunnels or plugging them with soft swab or other sterile gauze and selective drainage of the pleural space ought to be evaluated as alternatives to the present protocols. Can the obvious lack of retrospective data on acting otherwise provide arguments for keeping the status quo forever? Pierre Duval,[38] the father of French thoracic surgery, obtained very good results with a proactive attitude to indwelling objects almost 100 years ago.

Bony Structure Injuries Energy forces usually but not always are dissipated through the fractures of thoracic cage elements. Certain types of kinetic energies predispose to soft tissue injuries.[39] Indeed, 4% to 10% of all hospitalized trauma patients usually have associated rib fractures.[3] Rib fracture is one of the most frequent diagnoses at admission for trauma.[2,4] A review of post-traumatic rib fractures from a large series (548 cases; 39% of all admitted thoracic trauma) showed that isolated rib fractures were found in only in 13% of the total.[40] Pneumothorax, hemothorax or hemopneumothorax were noted in 396 (72.3%) of the cases with rib fracture requiring tube thoracostomy. Not surprisingly, the greater number of rib fractures. the higher morbidity, especially pulmonary, observed in more than 50% of the patients with more than five to six fractured ribs. Although the overall mortality for patients with rib fractures is reported to be around 6%, pulmonary complications can lead to death in 3.3% of these patients.[40]

Anterior and posterior axillary lines are predilection sites for costal injury.[14] Prognosis depends on the progress of the underlying lung. Proper pain relief, aggressive physiotherapy, incentive spirometry, and a semisitting position are still under-rated in the daily practice.

Some locations where rib fractures are encountered require special considerations.[40,41] In the event of fractures of the uppermost three ribs, the possibility of brachial plexus and thoracic outlet vascular injuries should be considered. Conversely, middle-zone fractures (ribs from third to eighth) need not to be underestimated, since 6% to 8% of rib fractures are bilateral, and multifocal fractures can easily compromise lung function on a longer run if pain relief or tracheobronchial toilette is insufficient. Advanced age, smoking, underlying lung pathologies (COPD), and low patient compliance are negative prognostic factors.

The plastron fracture pattern refers to the fracture of the costochondral junctions on either (or both) side(s) of the sternum. The presence of a concomitant sternal fracture may result in a paradoxical movement, rarely necessitating artificial ventilation or exceptionally osteosynthesis.

Potential liver, spleen, and kidney injuries should be ruled out in the event of fracture of the lowermost ribs (ninth and below). Diaphragmatic tears may coexist and demand surgical attention. Reportedly, lower thoracoabdominal stab wounds can hide a diaphragmatic injury in 15% to 20% of the cases, providing enough reason to consider elective video assisted thoracic surgery (VATS) exploration of the chest cavity if computed tomography (CT) image is doubtful.[42]

Chest wall implosion[43] lateral and lateroposterior multiple fractures represent an emerging entity on their own for causing serious deformity. Early nonendothoracic stabilization technique might prevent late complications and shorten hospital stay.

Fractured ribs may be driven inward, and lacerate lung parenchyma in turn may cause pneumothorax or with similar mechanism hemothorax. Detection of delayed hemopneumothorax requires repeated chest radiography within 48 to 72 hours of admission.

Fractures of the rib or other elements of the bony thorax often herald blunt intracavital trauma. It is important to notice that the absence of bony injuries does not exclude eventual major thoracic blunt trauma.[13,16,26,27] Fractures reflect the size and direction of energy that has been imparted to the thoracic wall, especially when scapulae and sternum are also involved. Therapy does not differ fundamentally from that of single rib fracture; only the degree of monitoring of the patient is higher. The main concern is the interference with ventilation via the Auer reflex.

Flail chest
Flail chest,[44,45] also known as stove-in[46] or crushed chest, occurs when a segment of at least four ribs fractures in two different places on the same side. The pathophysiology of flail chest has been described before.[47] Reportedly,

more than 75% of the flail chest injuries result from road traffic accidents, with mortality rates ranging between 5% and 36%.[48] In a large reported series of chest trauma reported from Israel, the incidence of flail chest was 2.2% (262 out of 11966 chest injuries), while the overall mortality reached 21% with increasing incidence for patients with advanced age and the significant injury severity score (ISS). Nevertheless, the occurrence of unilateral flail chest is not associated necessarily with an increased lethality.[48] Indeed, the more posterior and caudal this type of injury, the better the outcome. In almost 27% of these patients, flail chest was associated with severe brain injury.[26,48] Back in the mid 1970s, lung contusion, and not paradoxic chest wall movement, was recognized to be responsible for flail chest-related respiratory insufficiency.[49] The management of flail chest relies on two therapeutic approaches that are not mutually exclusive, namely the internal (or pneumatic) stabilization via artificial ventilation[50] and surgical reconstruction of chest wall stability.[47,51] A more conservative, lung injury-focused approach, addressed the intravascular fluid limitation, pain relief, and physiotherapy. Aggressive clearance of tracheobronchial secretions was preferred over ventilatory support. In this setting, epidural anesthesia decreased the incidence of pneumonia by about 45%.[44,49] Surgical stabilization of the chest wall was introduced by using wire stitches for broken ribs (1950), followed by intramedullary Rush nail fixation (1956).[3,4,47] Dynamic compression osteosynthesis with plates and bicortical screws has been considered as gold standard.[51] Controversy exists as to which outcome measure to consider, with survival as primary end point, and pneumonia, long-term disability, and procedure-specific complications as secondary ones. Recently, Athanassiadi and colleagues[52] identified the high ISS group as the most significant prognostic factor in a series of 250 flail chest injuries. In addition, the resorting to mechanical ventilation was not found to be necessary to achieve definitive treatment.[52]

Surgical treatment: osteosynthesis
There are four basic methods for osteosynthesis of broken ribs, developed mainly to treat flail chest, differentiated in their approach to the body of the rib.[3,46,47] External fixation may be accomplished by cerclage, using wiring/approximating stitches, which provides semirigid apposition of the injured part or using mesh in a carpet-like fashion. Vertical bridging belongs to this group, as the implants bridge the segment with the intact part of the thoracic cage. Use of Abrams rod, Nuss plates,

and derivatives, methyl-methacrylate (Palacos) prosthesis, and rib grafts has been reported.

Additionally, pericostal plates for osteosynthesis (Judet plate and its variations) may be used; these struts have different modifications in which the plate is provided with tongs to grasp the rib. The plates are usually made of metal, but absorbable materials are emerging, also.[53,54] The U-plate, follows a similar approach and needs extrapleural dissection only.

Intraosseal methods include intramedullary nailing and usage of pins. Combined methods have been reported as well, using plates with cerclage or bicortical screws. Locking screw might be useful, also.

Principles of surgical stabilization of broken ribs differ in their achieved degree of rigidity of the adjacent bone fragments and the role of the surrounding tissue. Biology-based dynamic approaches stemming from lung surgery favor anchoring methods in one camp, and bone axis-driven, time-honored osteosynthesis-centric orthopedic minds are for tight compression on the other. Those who have a strong orthopedic-based background tend to favor the rigid fixation. Both schools have strong arguments, and literature proves that both solutions are workable in their own context.[55] The permanent, 12–18/min frequency movement of the rib cage is a strong argument against stable fixation such as intramedullary device, screws, or plate application. Wire breakage, screw dislodgement, and consequent plate dislocation are not rare. Metal piece migration is a warning phenomenon, proving that foreign bodies cannot be left in situ indefinitely just to spare a second operation if they are otherwise accessible. Recent literature shows that surgical stabilization is gaining popularity in certain subset of flail chest patients. So far, two randomized studies with less than 100 cases in total are providing level 1 evidences.[45,56] Both papers suffer from a certain bias and are more than 5 years old, but the message, supported by nonrandomized cohort comparison series, sounds sensible, stating that a hazily defined subset of patients definitely benefit from surgery in terms of pneumonia and other respiration-related complications. There is a common methodological mistake, where days on ventilator are compared in the osteosynthesis groups to the pneumatic internal pneumatic stabilization one. In this tautologic analysis, osteosynthesis patients will be favored as one arm of the study contains the ventilated patients themselves. No paper refers to the time/discomfort, narcosis, and quality-of-life issues for a second surgery when the plates are to be removed.

While the jury remains out on whether surgical reconstruction of the noncontused lung subset of flail chest trauma patients is justified or not,[56] the next step is to define the appropriate timing of surgery. While the time window varies between 2 and 10 days,[43,45,56] elective chest wall reconstruction usually is preceded by keeping the patient on a ventilator in a hope of an early weaning. Careful selection of the fittest for surgery increases the chances for a favorable outcome, while ruling out those who would be unnecessarily operated on. The longer the waiting time, the better the results with surgery. While the heralding signs of a chest injury will call in due time for the need of respiratory support,[57] there is little to help in selecting those who can be weaned within a reasonable time and even less to help in identifying those who develop ventilator-related complications. The main causes of negative outcomes include tracheomalacia, post-intubation tracheal stricture, ventilator-related lung injury with the attendant colonization of multidrug-resistant species (eg, extended spectrum beta lactamase [ESBL]) producing Gram-negative bacteria and methicillin-resistant *Staphylococcus aureus* [MRSA]), and mycotic sepsis.[4,26,33]

Perioperative or prophylactic drainage are strongly recommended, as drainage is the sine qua non of pleural space control. Whenever positive end-expiratory pressure (PEEP) or continuous positive airway pressure (CPAP) ventilation is expected, a prophylactic thoracic drainage is the lesser evil, in spite of known probability of drainage complications.[58]

All in all, there are clear indications for osteosynthesis in order to restore chest wall stability (**Table 2**), even with minimally invasive methods (VATS).[59] Apart from fixation on the way out, when thoracotomy is performed for another reason, chest wall stabilization is justified for flail

Table 2 Surgical osteosynthesis for broken ribs			
Definite Yes	**+ +/-**	**+/- -**	**Definite No**
Thoracotomy for other reason	Flail chest Long posterior serial fracture	Severe deformity Severe pain	Severe lung contusion Brain injury

chest, which causes severe deformity, and exceptionally for intractable pain.[47,55,57] Questions about the best method for the osteosynthesis remain open, as no reliable comparative studies have been undertaken so far. One might say that the preference depending on the familiarity of the surgeon with a certain method is an acceptable basis for decision making, as there are no obviously inferior methods. However, whether all broken ribs with both ends of them be fixed or not, the practical answer is a definite no. Three re-unified pillar ribs are usually sufficient, and the moving window-like segment should be anchored to the rest of the cage.

The definite no surgery scenario is reserved for those with an utmost serious lung contusion as visualized by CT or proven otherwise.[47,57] However, the role of proper markers for biochemical monitoring of cell-level and subcellular lung injury remains to be clarified.

Sternum

Fractures of this massive spongious bone are either insignificant or associated with life-threatening conditions. They are typical injuries due to compression by steering wheel, dashboard, or direct blow. Patients with previous surgery in the chest region (open heart surgery, pectus anomaly) are prone to develop complicated fractures with serious complications. Most fractures occur in the upper third of the bone. Surgical stabilization is indicated only in case of serious dislocation, like significant over-riding or as a part of exploration for concomitant injuries (eg, heart or internal mammary injuries) on retreat. There are numerous sternum reconstruction methods, and the armamentarium (wire, compression plates) available is ample and the same as in any standard sternotomy.[60,61] The application of the Nuss procedure in a trauma scenario has been reported recently as a novel, minimally invasive method.[62] Prognosis is defined by the gravity of underlying injuries.

Shoulder blades

The importance of the fracture of the scapula lies mainly in predicting major intrathoracic injuries, as fracture of this massive bone is a good indicator of impartial energy.[4] The high-energy impact most commonly results in scattered fragments of the shattered scapula, implemented in the underlying lung parenchyma by the way. Scapular body osteosynthesis has anecdotal importance.

Clavicle

In up to one in five severe thoracic trauma patients, clavicular fracture presents as a secondary injury. Direct trauma (blow) and indirect injury (upper extremities) to the sternoclavicular junction can lead to sterile inflammation in the joint, causing a Tietze-like syndrome.[63] Locally administered anti-inflammatory therapy usually takes care of obstinate complaints. Resection of the painful syndesmosis without need for fixation is considered a last option. While fracture of the medial two thirds of the clavicle does not require stabilization, the involvement of the lateral third may call for osteosynthesis in order to achieve good girdle function.

Complex life-threatening injuries

There are two main reasons why complex serious blunt chest injuries show an absolute and relative increase within the general trauma profile. Passive defense measures increase the chance of survival for those who have suffered an upper torso injury, while asymmetric warfare (eg, improvised roadside devices) increase the frequency of these injuries.[4,8,12] In civilian scenarios, energy absorption zones and other active/passive defense (eg, seatbelts, air bags etc) measures implemented by the automotive industry may improve immediate survival chances. In the military new body armor may have the same effect. Closed-compartment blast injuries (either in an armed personnel carrier or a commuter train or school bus) have a common trauma profile.[8,22,64] Paradoxically, in these cases, the improved speed and efficacy of evacuation[65] along with the shortened time gaps in the infliction—care complex have worsened the overall survival statistics. In fact, more and more near-fatal cases, that formerly would have been dead on the spot, now arrive alive at the hospital. In military experience, penetrating bullet injuries are decreasing at expense of the increase of blast injuries, destroyed chest wall included.[66] Chest wall casualties are in a significant number among mass catastrophe sufferers, such as in earthquakes.[67] Sucking or blowing chest wounds[1] are extensive, full-thickness traumatic defects of the chest wall. They are caused by high-energy/velocity objects destroying the musculocutaneous and bony chest wall en masse. In military or civilian terror attack scenarios, the usual cause is the entry of an exploded irregularly shaped massive projectile or the exit of a yawing, tumbling smaller object, like a bullet.[8,12,22] Reportedly, 8% to 12% of all major thoracic casualties fall into this category. Immediate—accident/crime site/battlefield—treatment means cover the hole and drain the space. Airtight closure of the defect must be achieved in an improvised manner, using wide quadrangular bandage taped to the skin on three edges while leaving the fourth free in order to assure ventilating mechanisms. Asherman Chest Seal (Rusch, Tele-flex Medical Company, NC, USA) and Bolin Chest Seal (Combat Medical Systems, Fayetteville, NC, USA) devices are for emergency and immediate battlefield use for sucking chest wounds.[68] A pagoda roof-style bilayer multiholed bandage allows air escape at inhalation but closes during expiration. Definite treatment aims at the perma-nent cover for the underlying injured visceral pleura as soon as possible. Approximated or rotated adjacent autologous tissue provides the best cover. Securing viable, infection-free and well oxygenized/nutritioned tissue edges and tension-free approximation is essential, following a meticulous debridement. Anatomical resection of underlying lung after blunt chest injury is rarely indicated, as it occurs in under 1% of patients.[8,39] Lung-sparing techniques in form of tractotomy and stapled atypical resection are the standard.[11] Different biological seals,[69] autologous fibrin seal-ants, adhesive films,[70,71] and foam complexes[72,73] are recommended to cover troublesome lung surfaces and can also be applied for destroyed lung parenchyma. What chosen materials and methods have to fulfill in function is a more or less airtight covering of the lung parenchyma (prophylaxis of broncho/pneumopleural fistula (BPF/PPF) plus prevention of infection.[74] Systemic antibiotics and intelligent bandages play a supportive role, providing a cover for the rebuilt the integrity of the chest wall. Considering the reconstruction of the complex chest wall, there is a long list of well established methods. Synthetic meshes, polytetrafluoroethylene patches, and bovine pericardium are equally applied.[75,76] Appli-cation of longitudinally cut vascular prosthesis left-overs provides a good and budget-sensitive cover. Built-in metal plates and rods may add further stability to the complexes.[77] Usage of mesh-methyl-metacrylate sandwiches or Palacos alone, occasionally reinforced with built-in metal plates, are also reported.[78] Principles of chest wall reconstruction following oncologic resections are applied here also, with the caveat of the poten-tially infected environment. Nonautologous components are magnets for superinfection via colonization; as a consequence, bacteriological surveillance and antibiotic prophylaxis are of para-mount importance.[74] Infection control by vacuum-assisted closure device in the chest wall or in the underlying pleural space extended by drainage and evacuation (preferably by VATS) if needed, is to be initiated as soon as the first sign of insuffi-cient primary debridement emerges.[79]

Apart from implementing routine resuscitation measures, the most complete lung re-expansion should be the main concern of the surgeon. In this setting, extracorporeal lung support devices such as ECMO (extracorporeal membrane oxygenator) and pumpless lung assist systems represent signif-icant contributors in the management of chest wall injuries with extensive underlying parenchymal derangements. PICCO (pulse-induced continuous cardiac output) monitoring is invaluable in explosion-related penetrating injuries.[80] Combina-tion of explosions and burns from flash and hot gases in closed and confined areas causes burnt and blasted chest wall and lung. Blasted lung requires fluid restriction while, burned tissue requires ample volume replacement, making inten-sive therapy a tightrope walk. Sepsis, acute respi-ratory distress syndrome, and hepatorenal syndrome or insufficiency are the main complica-tions responsible for mortality, which can be as high as 60% to 80%, depending on the severity of other elements of polytrauma.

SUMMARY

Prognosis of chest wall injury depends mainly on the extent of underlying injuries (by lung paren-chyma and other organs). The golden hour rule will dominate the outcome, too, but most thoracic trauma cases is managed nonoperatively; even most surgical cases require chest drain alone. On the other hand, emergency thoracotomy for aortic or hilar cross-clamping—cardiac/great vessel wound control/stapling, or tractotomy do not need necessarily senior cardiothoracic surgeons. Critically ill, usually polytrauma patients will tolerate procedures only up to the point of an en masse stapled lung resection and temporary cover of extensive chest wall substance loss. The concept of thoracic damage control[10,11] includes both systemic and local hemorrhage control,[81] earliest repair of life-threatening tracheobronchial injuries, tractotomies, and tamponade of extensive lung lacerations. The best workforce scenario is to have surgeons at disposal with a good under-standing of the basics of thoracic surgery with a secondary line of those who are able to solve the complications (ie, specialists in cardiothoracic, plastic, and orthopedic surgery.

There is an opportunity to review the changes over the time gap of 20 years[82] since a similar review was published. The introduction of damage control and a multidisciplinary team approach to chest wall injury until the ventilated patient's condition would allow definite, usually combined plastic procedures are brand new elements. Oper-ative flail chest management is developing further and is gaining popularity due to changing trauma profiles (eg, mass terror attack casualties, asym-metric warfare, and refined explosion devices).

Due to an improved evacuation regime and advanced life support measures, thoracic surgeons nowadays participate in treatment of extensive chest injured patients never seen before to arrive alive. VACD provides a significant improvement in treatment efficacy of infected extensive chest wall injuries. A formerly existing gap in civilian and military surgical care philosophies in chest trauma is getting narrower, as there is much to learn from each other.[64] On the other side, in spite of new life support philosophies and devices, basic principles of chest wall trauma care have not changed dramatically.

ACKNOWLEDGMENTS

Laszlo Lukacs, MD, PhD, for his unselfish help in the preparation of this manuscript.

LTC Sandor Pellek, MD, for his invaluable advice on ongoing military surgical issues, North Atlantic Treaty Organization Military Medical Center of Excellence, Budapest, Hungary.

The late Tony Morgan, FRCS, my fellow-consultant at the Bristol Royal Infirmary, Bristol, United Kingdom, to whom I owe so much, not only for teaching me the behavior of the chest wall.

Veronika Martos—International Loan Services/ University of Pécs Medical Library—without whose help and contribution this manuscript would not have been realized.

REFERENCES

1. Nichols R. Casualty. The Wordsworth book of first world war poetry. Ware (UK): Wordworth Editions Ltd; 1995.
2. Demirhan R, Onan B, Oz K, et al. Comprehensive analysis of 4205 patients with chest trauma: a 10-year experience. Interact Cardiovasc Thorac Surg 2009;9:450−3.
3. Engel C, Krieg JC, Madey SM, et al. Operative chest wall fixation with osteosynthesis plates. J Trauma 2005;58:181−6.
4. Keel M, Meier C. Chest injuries—what is new? Curr Opin Crit Care 2007;13:674−9.
5. Smith N, Weymann D, Findlay G, et al. The management of trauma victims in England and Wales: a study by the National Confidential Enquiry into patient outcome and death. Eur J Cardiothorac Surg 2009;36(2):340−3.
6. Netscher DT, Baumholtz MA. Chest reconstruction: I. anterior and anterolateral chest wall and wounds affecting respiratory function. Plast Reconstr Surg 2009;124(5):240e−52e.
7. Weber PG, Huemmer HP, Reingruber B. Forces to be overcome in correction of pectus excavatum. J Thorac Cardiovasc Surg 2006;132(6):1369−73.
8. Propper BW, Gifford SM, Calhoon JH, et al. Wartime thoracic injury: perspectives in modern warfare. Ann Thorac Surg 2010;89(4):1032−5[discussion: 1035−6].
9. Aharonson-Daniel L, Klein Y, Peleg K. Suicide bombers form a new injury profile. Ann Surg 2006; 244:1018−23.
10. Beuran M, Iordache FM. Damage control surgery—new concept or reenacting of a classical idea? J Med Life 2008;1(3):247−53.
11. Rotondo MF, Bard MR. Damage control surgery for thoracic injuries. Injury 2004;35(7):649−54.
12. Biocina B, Sutlić Z, Husedzinović I, et al. Penetrating cardiothoracic war wounds. Eur J Cardiothorac Surg 1997;11(3):399−405.
13. Esme H, Solak O, Yurumez Y, et al. The prognostic importance of trauma scoring systems for blunt thoracic trauma. Thorac Cardiovasc Surg 2007;55 (3):190−5.
14. O'Connor JV, Adamski J. The diagnosis and treatment of noncardiac thoracic trauma. J R Army Med Corps 2010;156(1):5−14.
15. Karmy-Jones R, Jurkovich GJ. Blunt chest trauma. Curr Probl Surg 2004;41(3):211−380.
16. Avidan V, Hersch M, Armon Y, et al. Blast lung injury: clinical manifestations, treatment, and outcome. Am J Surg 2005;190:927−31.
17. Nishiumi N, Nakagawa T, Masuda R, et al. Endobronchial bleeding associated with blunt chest trauma treated by bronchial occlusion with a Univent. Ann Thorac Surg 2008;85(1):245−50.
18. Nishiumi N, Inokuchi S, Oiwa K, et al. Diagnosis and treatment of deep pulmonary laceration with intrathoracic hemorrhage from blunt trauma. Ann Thorac Surg 2010;89(1):232−8.
19. American College of Surgeons Committee on Trauma Advanced trauma Life Support (ATLS) for doctors; student course manual. 8th edition. Chicago: American College of Surgeons; 2007.
20. Nishiumi N, Maitani F, Tsurumi T, et al. Blunt chest trauma with deep pulmonary laceration. Ann Thorac Surg 2001;71(1):314−8.
21. Gayzik FS, Martin RS, Gabler HC. Characterization of crash-induced thoracic loading resulting in pulmonary contusion. J Trauma 2009;66(3):840−9.
22. Pizov R, Oppenheim-Eden A, Matot I, et al. Blast lung injury from an explosion on a civilian bus. Chest 1999;115:165−72.
23. Sasser SM, Sattin RW, Hunt RC, et al. Blast lung injury. Prehosp Emerg Care 2006;10(2):165−72.
24. Gill JR, Landi K. Traumatic asphyxial deaths due to an uncontrolled crowd. Am J Forensic Med Pathol 2004;25(4):358−61.
25. Noppen M, Verbanck S, Harvey J, et al. Music: a new cause of primary spontaneous pneumothorax. Thorax 2004;59:722−4.
26. Hildebrand F, Giannoudis PV, van Griensven M, et al. Management of polytraumatized patients

with associated blunt chest trauma: a comparison of two European countries. Injury 2005;36:293–302.

27. Onat S, Ulku R, Avci A, et al. Urgent thoracotomy for penetrating chest trauma: analysis of 158 patients of a single center. Injury 2010;41:876–80.

28. Molina DK, Wood LE, DiMaio VJ. Shotgun wounds: a review of range and location as pertaining to manner of death. Am J Forensic Med Pathol 2007; 28(2):99–102.

29. Degiannis E, Loogna P, Doll D, et al. Penetrating cardiac injuries: recent experience in South Africa. World J Surg 2006;30(7):1258–64.

30. Mattox KL. Prehospital care of the patient with and injured chest. Surg Clin North Am 1989;69:21–9.

31. Weyant MJ, Bains MS, Venkatraman E, et al. Results of chest wall resection and reconstruction with and without rigid prosthesis. Ann Thorac Surg 2006;81 (1):279–85.

32. McGillicuddy D, Rosen P. Diagnostic dilemmas and current controversies in blunt chest trauma. Emerg Med Clin North Am 2007;25(3):695–711.

33. Harrington DT, Phillips B, Machan J, et al. Factors associated with survival following blunt chest trauma in older patients: results from a large regional trauma cooperative [comment: 437–8]. Arch Surg 2010;145 (5):432–7.

34. Kelly S, Hughes S, Nixon S, et al. Spontaneous pneumomediastinum (Hamman's syndrome). Surgeon 2010;8(2):63–6.

35. Geusens E, Pans S, Van Breuseghem I, et al. Necrotizing fasciitis of the leg presenting with chest wall emphysema. Eur J Emerg Med 2004;11(1):49–51.

36. Ali HA, Lippmann M, Mundathaje U, et al. Spontaneous hemothorax: a comprehensive review. Chest 2008;134(5):1056–65.

37. Cothren CC, Moore EE. Emergency department thoracotomy for the critically injured patient: objectives, indications, and outcomes. World J Emerg Surg 2006;1:4.

38. Duval P. War wounds of the lung: notes on their surgical treatment at the front first English translation. Bristol (UK): Wyeth and Sons Limited; 1918.

39. Meredith JW, Hoth JJ. Thoracic trauma: when and how to intervene. Surg Clin North Am 2007;87: 95–118.

40. Sirmali M, Türüt H, Topçu S, et al. A comprehensive analysis of traumatic rib fractures: morbidity, mortality, and management. Eur J Cardiothorac Surg 2003;24(1):133–8.

41. Nirula R, Diaz JJ, Trunkey DD, et al. Rib fracture repair: indications, technical issues, and future directions. World J Surg 2009;33:14–22..

42. Bagheri R, Tavassoli A, Sadrizadeh A, et al. The role of thoracoscopy for the diagnosis of hidden diaphragmatic injuries in penetrating thoracoabdominal trauma. Interact Cardiovasc Thorac Surg 2009;9(2): 195–7 [discussion: 197–8].

43. Solberg BD, Moon CN, Nissim AA, et al. Treatment of chest wall implosion injuries without thoracotomy: technique and clinical outcomes. J Trauma 2009;67: 8–13.

44. Freedland M, Wilson RF, Bender JS, et al. The management of flail chest injury: factors affecting outcome. J Trauma 1990;30(12):1460–8.

45. Granetzny A, Abd El-Aal M, Emam E, et al. Surgical versus conservative treatment of flail chest. Evaluation of pulmonary status. Interact Cardiovasc Thorac Surg 2005;4:583–7.

46. Bloomer R, Willett K, Pallister I. The stove-in chest: a complex flail chest injury. Injury 2004;35(5):490–3.

47. Pettiford BL, Luketich JD, Landreneau RJ. The management of flail chest. Thorac Surg Clin 2007; 17(1):25–33.

48. Borman JB, Aharonson-Daniel L, Savitsky B, et al. Unilateral flail chest is seldom a lethal injury. Emerg Med J 2006;23(12):903–5.

49. Trinkle J, Richardson J, Franz J, et al. Management of flail chest without mechanical ventilation. Ann Thorac Surg 1975;19(4):355–63.

50. Avery EE, Morch ET, Benson DW. Critically crushed chests: new methods of treatment with continuous mechanical hyperventilation to produce alkalotic apnea and internal pneumatic stabilization. J Thorac Surg 1956;32:291–311.

51. París F, Tarazona V, Blasco E, et al. Surgical stabilization of traumatic flail chest. Thorax 1975;30:521–7.

52. Athanassiadi K, Theakos N, Kalantzi N, et al. Prognostic factors in flail chest patients. Eur J Cardiothorac Surg 2010;38(4):466–71.

53. Coonar AS, Qureshi N, Smith I, et al. A novel titanium rib bridge system for chest wall reconstruction. Ann Thorac Surg 2009;87:e46–8.

54. Mayberry JC, Terhes JT, Ellsi TJ, et al. Absorbable plates for rib fracture repair: preliminary experience. J Trauma 2003;55:835–9.

55. Mayberry JC, Ham LB, Schipper PH, et al. Surveyed opinion of American trauma, orthopedic, and thoracic surgeons on rib and sternal fracture repair. J Trauma 2009;66:875–9.

56. Tanaka H, Yukioka T, Yamaguti Y, et al. Surgical stabilization or internal pneumatic stabilization? A prospective randomized study of management of severe flail chest patients. J Trauma 2002;52: 727–32 [discussion: 732].

57. Voggenreiter G, Neudeck F, Aufinkolk M, et al. Operative chest wall stabilization in flail chest—outcomes of patients with or without pulmonary contusion. J Am Coll Surg 1998;187(2):130–8.

58. Harris A, O'Driscoll BR, Turkington PM. Survey of major complications of intercostal chest drain insertion in the UK. Postgrad Med J 2010;86(1012): 68–72.

59. Tagawa T, Itoh S, Ide S, et al. Repair of intrathoracic visceral damage using video-assisted thoracosocopic

surgery for blunt chest trauma and rib fixation at the site of minithoracotomy. Jpn J Thorac Cardiovasc Surg 1998;46:121–6.

60. Raman J, Straus D, Song DH. Rigid plate fixation of the sternum. Ann Thorac Surg 2007;84(3):1056–8.

61. Levin LS, Miller AS, Gajjar AH, et al. An innovative approach for sternal closure. Ann Thorac Surg 2010;89:1995–9.

62. Pacheco PE, Orem AR, Vegunta RK, et al. The novel use of Nuss bars for reconstruction of a massive flail chest. J Thorac Cardiovasc Surg 2009;138(5):1239–40.

63. Stochkendahl MJ, Christensen HW. Chest pain in focal musculoskeletal disorders. Med Clin North Am 2010;94(2):259–73.

64. Moore EE, Knudson MM, Schwab CW, et al. Military–civilian collaboration in trauma care and the senior visiting surgeon program. N Engl J Med 2007;357(26):2723–7.

65. Sanchez GP, Peng EW, Marks R, et al. Scoop and run strategy for a resuscitative sternotomy following unstable penetrating chest injury. Interact Cardiovasc Thorac Surg 2010;10(3):467–8.

66. Molnar TF, Hasse J, Jeyasingham K, et al. Changing dogmas: history of treatment for traumatic haemothorax pneumothorax and empyema thoracis. Ann Thorac Surg 2004;77:372–8.

67. Toker A, Isitmangh T, Erdik O, et al. Analysis of chest injuries sustained during the 1999 Marmara earthquake. Surg Today 2002;32:769–71.

68. Hodgetts TJ, Hanlan CG, Newey CG. Battlefield first aid: a simple, systematic approach for every soldier. J R Army Med Corps 1999;145(2):55–9.

69. Serra-Mitjans M, Belda-Sanchis J, Rami-Porta R. Surgical sealants for preventing air leaks after pulmonary resections in patients with lung cancer. Cochrane Database Syst Rev 2005;3:CD003051.

70. Anegg U, Lindenmann J, Matzi V, et al. Efficacy of fleece-bound sealing (Tachosil) of air leaks in lung surgery: a prospective randomised trial. Eur J Cardiothorac Surg 2007;31:198–202.

71. Transley P, Al-Mulhim F, Ladas G, et al. A prospective randomized controlled trial of the effectiveness of BioGlue in treating alveolar air leaks. J Thorac Cardiovasc Surg 2006;132:105–12.

72. Molnar TF, Farkas A, Stankovics J, et al. A new method for coping with lung parenchyma destruction in paediatric thoracic surgery. Eur J Cardiothorac Surg 2008;34(3):675–6.

73. Allen MS, Wood DE, Hawkinson RW, et al. Prospective randomized study evaluating a biodegradable polymeric sealant for sealing intraoperative air leaks that occur during pulmonary resection. Ann Thorac Surg 2004;77(5):1792–801.

74. Carbonell AM, Matthews BD, Deéau D, et al. The susceptibility of prosthetic biomaterials to infection. Surg Endosc 2005;19:430–5.

75. Shashidharan S, Karras R, Henry G. Use of Veritas acellular collagen matrix in chest wall reconstruction: an emerging choice. Am Surg 2010;76(2):218–20.

76. Wiegmann B, Zardo P, Dickgreber N, et al. Biological materials in chest wall reconstruction: initial experience with the Peri-Guard Repair Patch. Eur J Cardiothorac Surg 2010;37(3):602–5.

77. Lampl L. Chestwall resection: a new and simple method for stabilization of extended defects. Eur J Cardiothorac Surg 2001;20(4):669–73.

78. Molnar TF, Lukacs L, Horvath OP. Sternal replacement using composite allograft. Eur J Cardiothorac Surg 2002;21(2):371–3.

79. Palmen M, van Breugel HN, Geskes GG, et al. Open window thoracostomy treatment of empyema is accelerated by vacuum-assisted closure. Ann Thorac Surg 2009;88(4):1131–6.

80. Oren-Grinberg A. The PiCCO monitor. Int Anesthesiol Clin 2010;48(1):57–85.

81. Tien HCN, Gough MRC, Farrell R, et al. Successful use of recombinant activated coagulation factor VII in a patient with massive hemoptysis from a penetrating thoracic injury. Ann Thorac Surg 2007;84:1273–4.

82. Pate JW. Chest wall injuries in: thoracic trauma. Surg Clin North Am 1989;69(1):59–70.

Infections and Radiation Injuries Involving the Chest Wall

Justin D. Blasberg, MD[a], Jessica S. Donington, MD[b,c],*

KEYWORDS
- Chest wall • Necrosis • Infection • Radiation injury
- Resection

Soft tissue necrosis secondary to infection and radiation injury account for the majority of chest wall resections performed today that are unrelated to malignancy. Principles of treatment for chest wall infection and necrosis rely partially on the underlying cause and overall health of the patient but, in general, are based on wide resection of devitalized tissue and subsequent coverage with well vascularized and healthy soft tissue. Unlike most resection performed for malignancy, fibrosis of underlying tissues often precludes the need for skeletal reconstruction without loss of chest wall integrity or pulmonary function. Although the surgical management of these processes is similar, the underlying pathology differs significantly. Therefore, we address the risk factors, pathophysiology, clinical presentation, and management of chest wall infections and radiation injury separately.

CHEST WALL INFECTIONS

Infections of the chest wall are relatively uncommon but can be life threatening due to their negative impact on respiratory mechanics and potential for spread to the pleural space and mediastinum. Clinical outcome depends highly on the timing of intervention, severity of underlying, immune suppression, offending microbe, and extent of infection. Causative organisms include pyogenic bacteria, mycobacterium tuberculosis, and more unusual pathogens such as actinomycosis. The risk for chest wall infection is significantly increased by immune compromised states and a history of surgery or trauma to the region. In addition, patients with a history of intravenous drug use are at increased risk for developing septic arthritis of the sternoclavicular, sternochondral, and manubriosternal joints (**Fig. 1**).[1] In AIDS patients, chest wall infections tend to be more aggressive than those occurring in immune competent hosts and are associated with increased tissue destruction.[1]

Radiographic imaging plays an important role in the diagnosis of chest wall infection because clinical findings and laboratory tests can be unreliable, especially in the immune compromised patient. Chest radiograph is frequently the first imaging modality performed, but is often difficult to analyze. CT scanning and MRI are often complimentary in the diagnosis and quantification for extent of infection. A CT scan is more accurate at detecting bone destruction, whereas MRI provides better visualization of soft tissue involvement, which can be useful in preoperative planning. CT scan and ultrasound (US) may also be useful adjuncts, guiding percutaneous biopsies and drainage procedures.

[a] Department of General Surgery, St Luke's—Roosevelt Medical Center, Columbia University College of Physicians and Surgeons, 1000 Tenth Avenue, Suite 2B, New York, NY 10023, USA
[b] Department of Cardiothoracic Surgery, NYU School of Medicine, 530 1st Avenue, Suite 9V, New York, NY 10016, USA
[c] Department of Cardiothoracic Surgery, Bellevue Hospital, 462 First Avenue, New York, NY 10016, USA
* Corresponding author. Department of Cardiothoracic Surgery, NYU School of Medicine, 530 1st Avenue, Suite 9V, New York, NY 10016.
E-mail address: Jessica.donington@nyumc.org

Thorac Surg Clin 20 (2010) 487–494
doi:10.1016/j.thorsurg.2010.06.003
1547-4127/10/$ — see front matter © 2010 Elsevier Inc. All rights reserved.

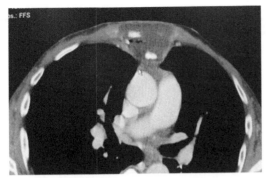

Fig. 1. Manubriosternal wound infection in a patient with long history of heroin use, admitted with persistent chest wall pain after minor trauma.

Sternoclavicular Joint Infection

The sternoclavicular joint is a gliding synovial joint with minimal soft tissue coverage. The joint includes the lateral notch of the manubrium, the medial inferior head of the clavicle, and the costocartilage of the first rib. Infections at the sternoclavicular joint represent only 2% of pyogenic arthritis. However, when present, they result in abscess formation in 20% of patients due to the joint capsule's inability to distend. Therefore, infection quickly spreads beyond the joint.[2] This often leads to fistula formation, abscesses, or mediastinitis. Predisposing factors for these infections include intravenous drug use and other immune compromised states such as diabetes, chronic hemodialysis, and longstanding steroid therapy, combined with local trauma or subclavian venous catheters.[3] Septic sternoclavicular joints have also been reported in women as a late complication of breast irradiation, typically 10 to 30 years after treatment following longstanding limitation of motion and skin changes.[2] Joint inoculation occurs most commonly by hematogenous spread, but can result from contiguous spread of infection. Responsible pathogens vary according to population; *Staphylococcus aureus* predominate in the general population, while *Pseudomonas aeruginosa* are frequently seen in intravenous drug users.[3] Thoracic surgeons are central in the management of these infections because of their proximity to the pleural space, mediastinum, and brachiocephalic structures.

Ninety-five percent of pyogenic sternoclavicular joint infections are unilateral, with a small predominance to the right side. Physical findings include focal tenderness, skin erythema, mild joint swelling, and induration over the affected joint.[4] Pain is a constant finding, but can be localized to the shoulder in up to 25% of patients, whereas fever occurs in only 65% of cases.[4] The median duration of symptoms at presentation is 14 days.[4] A classic presentation is demonstrated in a chronically immune suppressed patient who presents with unilateral chest or shoulder pain and a localized sternoclavicular mass or tenderness several weeks following a systemic illness.

Radiographic evaluation of sternoclavicular joint infections can be difficult. Plain radiographs and US are unreliable in the early phase of this infection. CT scanning is a superior diagnostic modality and the radiographic method of choice because of its spatial resolution in the chest wall. Bone erosion, sclerosis, and new bone formation are the radiographic hallmarks of this process and are well depicted on CT scan, but may not be visualized for 1 to 2 weeks following the onset of symptoms (**Fig. 2**). Late in the infectious process, plain radiographs alone can detect bony erosions and pseudo enlargement of the joint. In this setting, US is also useful for assessment of joint effusions, synovial enlargement, and associated soft tissue collections.[1]

Management of pyogenic septic arthritis is somewhat dependent on the extent of infection. An inflamed and indurated joint without evidence of bony destruction or extra capsular fluid can initially be managed conservatively with removal of any potential seeding source (ie, central venous

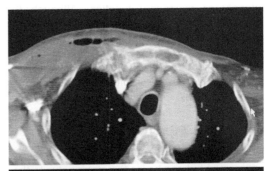

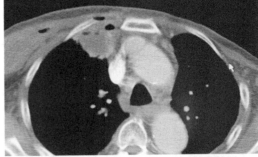

Fig. 2. CT scan of a right-sided sternoclavicular joint infection. Scan demonstrates bone destruction, capsular thickening, and extra capsular fluid collections on the overlying chest wall and underside of the joint.

catheter) and broad-spectrum intravenous antibiotics. Incision and drainage has been reported to be useful in cases with limited disease or when a specimen for histopathologic examination is required for diagnosis.[4] If a less invasive approach is used for control of an early infection, close follow-up is mandatory because resolution of this process following simple incision and drainage is relatively uncommon.[3,5] Failure to control infection by incision and drainage mandates aggressive surgical debridement for adequate treatment. The presence of a periarticular fluid collection, abscess, bony destruction, or persistent infection following antibiotic therapy are additional indications for surgery, which can be performed either as a wide en bloc resection of the joint and involved tissues, or as piece meal debridement of non-viable structures.

Formal en bloc joint resection or piecemeal debridement are both typically performed via an inverted L- shaped incision that extends laterally over the medial half of the clavicle and inferiorly over the manubrium down to the second or third interspace. Devitalized soft tissue is widely debrided and viable pectoralis and sternocleidomastoid muscle fibers are resected away from the bony structures and areas of phlegmon. A Rongeur is typically used to debride necrotic bone, infected joint material, and to access abscess cavities. When formal en-bloc joint resection is performed, a periosteal elevator is used to separate soft tissues from areas of bony division. A Gigli saw is typically used to divide the clavicle 2 to 3 cm lateral to the inflammatory mass. The manubrium may be divided with a Lebski knife or sternal saw. However, only half the manubrium is typically resected to preserve stability of the contralateral side. The costal cartilage and medial portion of the first rib can then be divided with rib instruments, along with medial portions of the second or third rib if involved with infection. Concomitant resection of the great vessels is not typically indicated and injury to vascular structures was not reported in the two largest surgical series to date.[3,5] Sternoclavicular infections frequently require serial operative debridements to ensure adequate removal of all infected and devitalized tissue before closure. Open wounds can be packed with gauze or a vacuum-assisted closure (VAC) device (KCI, San Antonio, TX, USA) can be placed between procedures. Small defects can be left to heal by secondary intention. However, the majority of wounds require soft tissue coverage for closure—most commonly accomplished with an ipsilateral pectoralis muscle advancement flap.[3,5] Long-term antibiotics are usually required in conjunction with aggressive surgical treatment

when severe infection is present. Despite the aggressive nature of debridement required to eradicate sternoclavicular joint infections, postoperative shoulder function is usually preserved and the majority of patients report normal upper extremity performance at long-term follow-up.[3,5]

The largest series of sternoclavicular joint infections treated by surgery was reported by Burkhart and colleagues[5] from the Mayo Clinic. In their series of 26 patients, pain was the most commonly reported symptom followed by swelling over the joint. Half of the patients evaluated had a recent or ongoing systemic infection and five had a history of trauma. Four patients had undergone previous incision and drainage, and wound cultures were positive in nearly all patients. Unilateral debridement was most commonly performed making use of an ipsilateral pectoralis muscle flap for closure. Patients received antibiotics for a median of 42 days following surgery.

Atypical infection can also occur at the sternoclavicular joint: approximately 3% of extraspinal tuberculosis arthritis occur at this location.[6] Radiographic characteristics unique to tuberculosis infections include an inflammatory mass, absence of new bone formation, and calcifications in the abscess wall, which can also be associated with compression of the subclavian vessels by the inflammatory mass. Histologic or microbiologic evaluation is necessary to obtain a definitive diagnosis.

Brucellar sternoclavicular arthritis is a rare but classically described pathology.[7] Brucellosis is a naturally occurring gram-negative, facultative pathogen in domesticated animals. Human infections occur through consumption of infected raw meat and milk products in endemic areas such as the Mediterranean, Middle East, Latin America, and Asia. Human brucellosis is a multisystem disease, but most patients present with musculoskeletal involvement. The sternoclavicular joint is a lesser involved location (2%–5%).[8] Diagnosis requires microbiological confirmation of the organism or demonstration of antibodies by serologic testing. Treatment requires 6 to 12 weeks of a two-drug regime with streptomycin and doxycycline or tetracycline to eradicate the organism from bone.[8] Surgical intervention is almost never indicated with sternoclavicular involvement.

An important differential to consider for the diagnoses of pyogenic sternoclavicular joint infections is SAPHO (synovitis, acne, pustulosis, hyperostosis, and osteitis) syndrome. This complex set of musculoskeletal disorders and associated skin conditions, first described by Hayem and colleagues[9] in 1987, is defined by joint and skin inflammatory processes in the absence of infectious cause. SAPHO syndrome is well known by rheumatologists and dermatologists. Yet is is relatively unknown to thoracic surgeons, despite the fact that the sternoclavicular joint is the most common site of skeletal involvement—seen in 63% to 90% of cases. This syndrome occurs most commonly in adolescents and young adults, and usually follows a prolonged relapsing course. Bone pain as a result of hyperostosis and osteitis is the most prominent and troublesome symptom. CT scan and MRI are of little utility in differentiating this disease from pyogenic arthritis, but bone scan can be useful in detecting a pattern of involvement typical of SAPHO with inflammation at the sternoclavicular joint, sacroiliac joint, and spine. Osteitis in SAPHO is a result of sterile inflammatory infiltrates, and cultures from joint aspirations and bone biopsies are usually negative.[9] In an otherwise healthy young adult who presents with recurrent sternoclavicular arthritis and no clear history of immune suppression or infectious cause, a careful history for associated skin disorders is important. Patients diagnosed with SAPHO have frequently undergone long courses of unnecessary antibiotics and surgical debridements only to incur disease relapse. The primary treatment for SAPHO involves NSAIDs. This is usually accompanied by antimicrobial therapy against Propionibacterium acnes, a low virulence agent, isolated in a handful of cases.[9] If symptoms persist following 4 weeks of NSAIDs therapy, a trial of bisphosphonates and more aggressive anti-inflammatory agents are added. Surgery is only indicated when bone mechanics are adversely effected by the inflammation, which is more common with spine and long-bone involvement than the sternoclavicular joint.[10]

Necrotizing Chest Wall Infections

Necrotizing soft tissue infections are a highly aggressive and lethal subset of infections that require early and aggressive surgical intervention. These infections occur most commonly on the abdomen, perineum, and lower extremities, but can occur at any location, including the chest wall. The incidence of necrotizing infections is higher in immune compromised populations, particularly diabetics.[11–13] Patients typically present with pain out of proportion to the wound's clinical appearance and wound features, including erythema, swelling, skin blistering, crepitus, and watery drainage, are often present. Systemic evidence of infection includes fever, chills, mental status changes, hypotension, and tachycardia. It is useful to view necrotizing infections as a spectrum of clinical conditions with a similar pathologic condition. A small percentage of these infections are caused by a single organism, such as Clostridium perfringens or Streptococcus species. More typically, however, necrotizing infections are polymicrobial with both aerobic and anaerobic bacteria. These organisms work synergistically to produce fulminate infection and necrosis, which typically occurs in proximity to a surgical procedure such as chest tube placement for empyema drainage.[12,13]

Treatment of necrotizing soft tissue infection of the chest wall is the same as for necrotizing infection at other locations and includes early and aggressive surgical debridement, broad spectrum antibiotic therapy, fluid resuscitation, and cardiopulmonary support to maintain end-organ perfusion. Patients often require daily operative debridements of the infectious source control. Necrotizing infections of the chest wall can be complicated by pleural space involvement and respiratory impairment, which may account for the very high associated mortality (59%—89%), approximately twice that of similar infections at other anatomic locations.[11,13] When debridement is complete, all devitalized tissue has been removed, and patients are hemodynamically stable, skeletal reconstruction is usually required and may be technically challenging. The rapid onset of these infections does not allow for the development of underlying fibrosis. In addition, these defects tend to be large and some restoration of chest wall structural integrity is often required to reduce ventilator requirements. Use of prosthetic mesh is contraindicated due to infectious risk, thus cadaveric skin has become an attractive option for skeletal reconstruction. Soft tissue coverage is also required with chest wall reconstruction; this can be technically challenging due to the large size of the defect and frequent, involvement of the chest wall muscles most commonly used for tissue flaps.

Infections Secondary to Tuberculosis and Other Atypical Pathogens

The chest wall is an unusual location for tuberculosis infections. Extra pulmonary infections account for only 15% to 20% of all tuberculosis infections, and infections involving the chest wall account for only 10% of those.[14] However, widespread proliferation of HIV is thought to be responsible for the dramatic resurgence of tuberculosis in the past decade.[15] Tuberculosis abscesses of the chest wall can involve the ribs, costochondral junctions, costovertebral joints, and the vertebrae, but have a strong predilection for the margins of the sternum. It is hypothesized that infections at this location result from internal mammary lymph node infections that develop secondary to pulmonary involvement. The lymph nodes then caseate and erode through the chest wall, resulting in visible swelling. Subpleural collections of caseous material from necrosed lymph nodes are referred to as "cold abscesses." Subsequent erosion of bone by tuberculosis results from either pressure necrosis by granulation tissue or as a direct result of bone infection by the organism. Once a tuberculosis diagnosis is established systemic multidrug therapy is the mainstay of therapy.[16] However, cold abscess of the chest wall due to tuberculosis usually require surgical resection, because medical treatment alone is not adequate.[17,18] Wide excision and aggressive debridement of infected soft tissue and the bone chest wall is required to prevent recurrence. Reconstruction with muscle flap is typically required.

Thoracic actinomycosis is another rare cause of chest wall infection. The causative agent, is a gram-positive anaerobic bacteria found in the oral flora of healthy humans. Infection occurs with disruption of the normal mucosal barrier and spread of the bacteria into previously sterile body sites. There are three major forms of actinomycosis: cervicofacial (65%), abdominal (20%), and thoracic (15%).[19] Thoracic infections usually occur as a result of aspiration in a patient with poor oral hygiene, and usually originate in the lung parenchyma and can progress through the pleura to the chest wall. Thoracic actinomycosis may be complicated by empyema, hemoptysis, chronic draining sinus, and systemic dissemination.[20] Actinomycosis infections limited to the chest wall, without evidence of pulmonary involvement are rare but has been reported and can be easily confused with a primary chest wall tumor.[19] Diagnosis is made by isolating *Actinomyces* from normally sterile body sites, but the organism is difficult to grow in culture media. Therefore, diagnosis often requires surgical biopsy and histopathologic examination for the presence of grainy microcolonies of the organism, the so-called "sulfur granules" that are hallmark of the disease. Treatment includes incision and drainage of affected areas and long-term penicillin therapy.[21]

RADIATION INJURY TO THE CHEST WALL

Radiation therapy is a well-established treatment modality for a wide range of malignancies. It is estimated that 50% of the 1,200,000 new cases of cancer diagnosed each year in the United States will receive radiation, and 50% of those will be long-term survivors.[22] The main therapeutic action of radiation is via induction of toxic oxidative damage in targeted cells through alterations of mitochondrial membrane potential and mitochondrial-dependant generation of reactive oxygen species. Excessive production of reactive oxygen species leads to increased oxidative stress, damage to intercellular organelles, and ultimately necrosis. Radiation inevitably results in injury to normal tissue in the path of therapy, but these acute normal tissue changes generally resolve with the completion of therapy. Serious complications that occur months to years after treatment, collectively known as late radiation tissue injury (LRTI), occur in 5% to 15% of long-term survivors and vary significantly with age, dose, and site of treatment.[23–25] There appears to be an increase in number of LTRI from earlier treatment approaches which accompanies the increasing prevalence of long-term cancer survivors. It is becoming increasingly evident that as we increase our ability to provide definitive curative therapy to patients, avoidance of LTRI is of greater importance because of its significant negative impact on patient quality of life.

LTRI is characterized by a progressive deterioration of tissue secondary to reduced vascularity, due primarily to decreased density and obliteration of tissue-related small vessels. This is followed by replacement of normal soft tissue architecture by dense fibrotic tissue until there is insufficient oxygen delivery to sustain normal function. The cellular and molecular mechanisms of late radiation fibrosis are due to an abnormal interaction between fibroblasts and transforming growth factor beta (TGF-β), resulting in aberrant fibroblast proliferation, early terminal differentiation of fibroblasts, and a several-fold increase in the synthesis and deposition of collagen. Atypical "radiation" fibroblasts are large, triangle-shaped cells that are characteristically involved in LTRI.[26] LTRI is also characterized by a paucity of cellular inflammatory response with a near complete lack of granulocytes, lymphocytes, and macrophages in the effected stroma. Progressive tissue damage continues until a critical point when tissue down results in ulceration or an area with a confluence of cell death recognized as radiation necrosis.[27]

Although LTRI can occur in any tissue, it is most commonly seen in the head and neck, chest wall, and pelvis, reflecting the anatomic locations most commonly irradiated and those malignancies with a high likelihood of survival. Breast malignancies are the most common reason for chest wall radiation. External beam radiation has been one of the pillars of breast cancer therapy over the past decade due to increased use of breast-conserving surgery with radiotherapy for early stage disease. Radiation to the chest wall is associated with an increased risk for spontaneous rib fractures and skeletal side effects partially due to combination with hormonal and chemotherapeutic agents, which significantly decrease bone mineral density.[28] The spectrum of LTRI following treatment for breast cancer is quite heterogeneous, ranging from breast hyperpigmentation, skin dryness, chronic edema, and telangiectasias to pulmonary fibrosis, chronic ulceration, spontaneous rib fractures, fat necrosis, osteonecrosis, and neurologic disorders secondary to perineural fibrosis.[29]

Hyperbaric oxygen therapy has been proposed as a treatment modality that can improve tissue quality and prevent tissue breakdown in irradiated areas. It is defined by the administration of 100% oxygen at an environment pressure greater than atmospheric, which increases the pressure of oxygen delivered to the lungs and blood. Patients are placed in an airtight vessel and given 100% oxygen to breathe while atmospheric pressure is raised to 2.0 to 2.5 atmospheres for a period of 1 to 2 hours. Treatment is typically provided once or twice daily for up to 60 sessions. Hyperbaric oxygen therapy has been shown to increase the density of blood vessels in irradiated tissue in both animal and human models.[30] It is used most extensively for LTRI of the mandible, head and neck, and rectum or anus.[31] In addition, there are a handful of series reporting benefit to injuries of the chest wall following breast irradiation.[32–35] Hyperbaric oxygen therapy decreased the lesser extent of LTRI including chronic breast edema, induration and pain,[33] as well as reducing the severity of skin, soft tissue and bone necrosis.[36] Hyperbaric oxygen therapy has also been used as an adjunct to surgery to improve the likelihood of skin graft survival at this location.[35]

When LTRI of the chest wall progresses to skin breakdown and ulceration, biopsy is always required to rule out recurrence of the primary tumor or a radiation-induced squamous cell carcinoma or soft tissue sarcoma.[37] Women exposed to radiotherapy are at a fourfold increased risk for the development of sarcoma to the chest wall or arm, the majority of which appear after a 10 to 12 year latency.[38] Radiation-associated chest wall wounds pose a significant health hazard because of the impediment to normal respiratory function and the risk of infectious spread to the pleural space. These injuries typically involve the anterior aspect of the third, fourth, and fifth ribs.[38] The principles of management once malignancy has been ruled out include debridement of necrotic tissues and reconstruction with well-vascularized flaps.

The goals of treatment are to palliate symptoms and prevent spread of infection to the intrathoracic space, but there are numerous controversies regarding the practical management of LTRI patients. Most surround the appropriate timing and extent of resection, utility of hyperbaric oxygen to reduce symptoms and improve tissue quality, and the use of prosthetic materials in a contaminated field. The negative impact of these wounds on the patient's quality of the life is an incredibly important consideration when determining the timing of surgical intervention. The extent of resection, often involving subtotal chest wall excision, can be associated with significant postoperative morbidity and lengthy periods of recovery. Therefore, proper and careful surgical technique is imperative for appropriate healing and to prevent wound breakdown.

Once all necrotic or tumor-bearing tissue has been fully removed, healthy vascularized tissue coverage is most commonly supplied by myocutaneous rotational flaps from the pectoralis, latissimus dorsi, or rectus abdominis muscles. The omentum has also been used with excellent results, but requires laparoscopy or laparotomy for harvest and coverage with a skin graft.[39] Radiation to the blood supply of a myocutaneous flap is not a contraindication to use because large vessels are not typically affected by therapy. Because excessive fibrosis is one of the hallmarks of LTRI, the majority of LTRI wounds, even when full thickness, do not require skeletal reconstruction with synthetic mesh before the placement of the muscle flaps. The underling fibrosis and bulk of the muscle flap provide adequate chest wall rigidity. However, in the immediate postoperative period, these patients can suffer from paradoxical chest wall movement during respiration that may require a brief period of mechanical ventilation. This typically resolves over days without any long-term compromise of respiratory mechanics or pulmonary function.[37] Mesh reconstruction may be considered when omentum and a skin graft are used over a large area on the lateral chest wall.[39]

VACUUM-ASSISTED CLOSURE TECHNOLOGY

Infected and radiation-induced wounds can be a difficult to manage. The complexities are magnified for wounds on the chest wall because of their proximity to the pleural space and associated impact on respiratory mechanics. Vacuum-assisted closure (VAC) technology has proven to be a very effective tool in the management of complex chest wall wounds.[40] Subatmospheric pressure dressings are now commercially available as the VAC device (KCI, San Antonio, TX, USA). VACs are an incredibly effective method to accelerate wound healing by maintaining an optimal environment with subatmospheric pressure at approximately 125 mm Hg with an alternating cycle of 5 minutes on suction followed by 2 minutes off suction. Animal studies have demonstrated that this regime increases blood flow, decreases tissue edema, removes excessive fluid from the wound bed, and facilitates the removal of bacteria.[41] Subatmospheric pressure also alters the cytoskeleton of the cells in the wound bed and triggers a cascade of intracellular signals that increase cell division and subsequent formation of granulation tissue.[42] These effects make the VAC device an extremely versatile tool in the wound healing armamentarium.

The VAC device has a wide range of clinical applications, including treatment of infected surgical wounds, traumatic wounds, pressure ulcers, wounds with exposed bone and hardware, diabetic foot ulcers, venous stasis ulcers, and tissue breakdown associated with radiation. VAC use for LTRI wounds of the chest wall has been shown to decrease the number of operative debridements, shorten hospital stays, decrease rates of infection, and increase the rate of primary wound closure.[43] VACs have been safely used following thoracotomy or within the pleural space to control complicated wounds with an associated pleural component. Additionally, they can be safely and easily used in the outpatient setting, allowing for resumption of daily activities and elective planning of a definitive reconstructive procedure. VACs are generally well tolerated, with few contraindications or complications, and have quickly become a mainstay of current wound care.

SUMMARY

Necrotic and pyogenic chest wall wounds are relatively rare, but more common in immune-compromised patients and those with underlying trauma, surgery, or chest wall irradiation. Aggressive surgical debridement of all infected and devitalized tissue followed with coverage by well vascularized soft tissue is the mainstay of therapy regardless of the underlying cause. These wounds and infections carry increased morbidity and mortality compared with their counterparts at other anatomic locations because of the risk of infectious spread into the pleural space and mediastinum. In addition, they negatively impact the patient's normal respiratory mechanics and overall quality of life. The VAC device, which removes infectious materials and stimulates granulation, has become an important management adjunct to wide debridement and muscle flap reconstruction for these complex wounds.

REFERENCES

1. Chelli Bouaziz M, Jelassi H, Chaabane S, et al. Imaging of chest wall infections. Skeletal Radiol 2009;38(12):1127–35.
2. Chanet V, Soubrier M, Ristori JM, et al. Septic arthritis as a late complication of carcinoma of the breast. Rheumatology (Oxford) 2005;44(9):1157–60.
3. Song HK, Guy TS, Kaiser LR, et al. Current presentation and optimal surgical management of sternoclavicular joint infections. Ann Thorac Surg 2002;73(2):427–31.
4. Ross JJ, Shamsuddin H. Sternoclavicular septic arthritis: review of 180 cases. Medicine (Baltimore) 2004;83(3):139–48.
5. Burkhart HM, Deschamps C, Allen MS, et al. Surgical management of sternoclavicular joint infections. J Thorac Cardiovasc Surg 2003;125(4):945–9.
6. Adler BD, Padley SP, Muller NL. Tuberculosis of the chest wall: CT findings. J Comput Assist Tomogr 1993;17(2):271–3.
7. Alton GG, Jones LM, Pietz DE. Laboratory techniques in brucellosis. Monogr Ser World Health Organ 1975;55:1–163.
8. Geyik MF, Gur A, Nas K, et al. Musculoskeletal involvement of brucellosis in different age groups: a study of 195 cases. Swiss Med Wkly 2002;132(7–8):98–105.
9. Hayem G, Bouchaud-Chabot A, Benali K, et al. SAPHO syndrome: a long-term follow-up study of 120 cases. Semin Arthritis Rheum 1999;29(3):159–71.
10. Matzaroglou C, Velissaris D, Karageorgos A, et al. SAPHO syndrome diagnosis and treatment: report of five cases and review of the literature. Open Orthop J 2009;3:100–6.
11. Praba-Egge AD, Lanning D, Broderick TJ, et al. Necrotizing fasciitis of the chest and abdominal wall arising from an empyema. J Trauma 2004;56(6):1356–61.
12. Safran DB, Sullivan WG. Necrotizing fasciitis of the chest wall. Ann Thorac Surg 2001;72(4):1362–4.
13. Urschel JD, Takita H, Antkowiak JG. Necrotizing soft tissue infections of the chest wall. Ann Thorac Surg 1997;64(1):276–9.
14. Mathlouthi A, Ben M'Rad S, Merai S, et al. [Tuberculosis of the thoracic wall. Presentation of 4 personal cases and review of the literature]. Rev Pneumol Clin 1998;54(4):182–6 [in French].
15. Condos R, Rom WN, Weiden M. Lung-specific immune response in tuberculosis. Int J Tuberc Lung Dis 2000;4(2 Suppl 1):S11–7.

16. Jain S, Shrivastava A, Chandra D. Breast lump, a rare presentation of costochondral junction tuberculosis: a case report. Cases J 2009;2:7039.

17. Cho S, Lee EB. Surgical resection of chest wall tuberculosis. Thorac Cardiovasc Surg 2009;57(8):480–3.

18. Lim SY, Pyon JK, Mun GH, et al. Reconstructive surgical treatment of tuberculosis abscess in the chest wall. Ann Plast Surg 2010;64(3):302–6.

19. Chernihovski A, Loberant N, Cohen I, et al. Chest wall actinomycosis. Isr Med Assoc J 2007;9(9):686–7.

20. Mabeza GF, Macfarlane J. Pulmonary actinomycosis. Eur Respir J 2003;21(3):545–51.

21. Bennhoff DF. Actinomycosis: diagnostic and therapeutic considerations and a review of 32 cases. Laryngoscope 1984;94(9):1198–217.

22. Jemal A, Siegel R, Ward E, et al. Cancer statistics, 2009. CA Cancer J Clin 2009;59(4):225–49.

23. Stone HB, Coleman CN, Anscher MS, et al. Effects of radiation on normal tissue: consequences and mechanisms. Lancet Oncol 2003;4(9):529–36.

24. Thompson IM, Middleton RG, Optenberg SA, et al. Have complication rates decreased after treatment for localized prostate cancer? J Urol 1999;162(1): 107–12.

25. Waddell BE, Rodriguez-Bigas MA, Lee RJ, et al. Prevention of chronic radiation enteritis. J Am Coll Surg 1999;189(6):611–24.

26. Fajardo LF. The pathology of ionizing radiation as defined by morphologic patterns. Acta Oncol 2005;44(1):13–22.

27. Rodemann HP, Bamberg M. Cellular basis of radiation-induced fibrosis. Radiother Oncol 1995; 35(2):83–90.

28. Hirbe A, Morgan EA, Uluckan O, et al. Skeletal complications of breast cancer therapies. Clin Cancer Res 2006;12(20 Pt 2):6309S–14S.

29. Fehlauer F, Tribius S, Holler U, et al. Long-term radiation sequelae after breast-conserving therapy in women with early-stage breast cancer: an observational study using the LENT-SOMA scoring system. Int J Radiat Oncol Biol Phys 2003;55(3):651–8.

30. Marx RE, Ehler WJ, Tayapongsak P, et al. Relationship of oxygen dose to angiogenesis induction in irradiated tissue. Am J Surg 1990;160(5):519–24.

31. Bennett M, Feldmeier J, Smee R, et al. Hyperbaric oxygenation for tumour sensitisation to radiotherapy: a systematic review of randomised controlled trials. Cancer Treat Rev 2008;34(7):577–91.

32. Feldmeier JJ. Hyperbaric oxygen for delayed radiation injuries. Undersea Hyperb Med 2004;31(1): 133–45.

33. Carl UM, Feldmeier JJ, Schmitt G, et al. Hyperbaric oxygen therapy for late sequelae in women receiving radiation after breast-conserving surgery. Int J Radiat Oncol Biol Phys 2001;49(4):1029–31.

34. Carl UM, Hartmann KA. Hyperbaric oxygen treatment for symptomatic breast edema after radiation therapy. Undersea Hyperb Med 1998;25(4):233–4.

35. Hart GB, Mainous EG. The treatment of radiation necrosis with hyperbaric oxygen (OHP). Cancer 1976;37(6):2580–5.

36. Feldmeier JJ, Heimbach RD, Davolt DA, et al. Hyperbaric oxygen as an adjunctive treatment for delayed radiation injury of the chest wall: a retrospective review of twenty-three cases. Undersea Hyperb Med 1995;22(4):383–93.

37. Granick MS, Larson DL, Solomon MP. Radiation-related wounds of the chest wall. Clin Plast Surg 1993;20(3):559–71.

38. Senkus-Konefka E, Jassem J. Complications of breast-cancer radiotherapy. Clin Oncol (R Coll Radiol) 2006;18(3):229–35.

39. Sato M, Tanaka F, Wada H. Treatment of necrotic infection on the anterior chest wall secondary to mastectomy and postoperative radiotherapy by the application of omentum and mesh skin grafting: report of a case. Surg Today 2002;32(3):261–3.

40. Welvaart WN, Oosterhuis JW, Paul MA. Negative pressure dressing for radiation-associated wound dehiscence after posterolateral thoracotomy. Interact Cardiovasc Thorac Surg 2009;8(5):558–9.

41. Morykwas MJ, Simpson J, Punger K, et al. Vacuum-assisted closure: state of basic research and physiologic foundation. Plast Reconstr Surg 2006;117 (Suppl 7):121S–6S.

42. Saxena V, Hwang CW, Huang S, et al. Vacuum-assisted closure: microdeformations of wounds and cell proliferation. Plast Reconstr Surg 2004; 114(5):1086–96 [discussion: 1097–8].

43. Siegel HJ, Long JL, Watson KM, et al. Vacuum-assisted closure for radiation-associated wound complications. J Surg Oncol 2007;96(7):575–82.

Primary Chest Wall Tumors

Shona E. Smith, MD, FRCSC[a],
Shaf Keshavjee, MD, MSc, FRCSC[a,b],*

KEYWORDS

- Chest wall tumors • Chest wall sarcoma • Ewing sarcoma
- Chondrosarcoma • Osteosarcoma

INTRODUCTION

Patients with chest wall tumors present diagnostic and therapeutic challenges. The differential diagnosis of these tumors is broad, because they can represent a heterogeneous spectrum of diseases from primary benign or malignant tumors to metastases; local extension of adjacent tumors of the lung, mediastinum, pleura or breast; non-neoplastic infectious or inflammatory conditions; or even local manifestations of systemic disease. Primary chest wall tumors are best classified according to their tissue of origin, bone or soft tissue, and further subclassified according to whether or not they are benign or malignant. Most of these tumors are uncommon, with information garnered from individual case reports or institutional case series.

Chest wall tumors are more commonly either metastases or local invasion of an underlying adjacent tumor. Primary chest wall tumors account for only 0.04% of all new cancers diagnosed and 5% of all thoracic neoplasms.[1] The list of potential tumors is broad (**Table 1**), with nomenclature that is frequently overlapping and sometimes contradictory in the literature. Primary benign lesions of the chest wall can behave in a latent, active, or aggressive manner. Approximately 60% of primary chest wall tumors are malignant. Although primary chest wall tumors are diagnosed in every age group, they are more likely malignant in the extremes of age: in the young and the elderly. Certain tumors present predominantly in one age group. For example, Ewing sarcoma is more common in children and young adults, primitive neuroectodermal tumor (PNET) in patients in their 20s, and chondrosarcoma in middle adult life and solitary plasmacytoma occurs more frequently in older adults. Of malignant tumors, chondrosarcoma and lymphoma are most prominent in adults,[2] whereas in children, Ewing sarcoma and rhabdomyosarcoma are the most common tumors.[3]

DIAGNOSIS

Patients often present with a palpable enlarging mass. Less commonly, asymptomatic patients are diagnosed due to an incidental finding on imaging as part of screening or for investigation of an unrelated condition. Soft tissue masses are often painless, whereas bony lesions, both benign and malignant, are typically painful due to growth and periosteal damage. Symptoms develop as the tumor grows and can be associated with local invasion of adjacent structures. Paresthesias and weakness may be present if neurologic structures, such as the spinal cord or brachial plexus, are involved. Systemic symptoms of fever, malaise, fatigue, and weight loss in addition to suggesting infection or metastasis, are also seen in eosinophilic granuloma and Ewing sarcoma. Due to the rarity of chest wall tumors, the time between onset of symptoms and diagnosis is often long.[4] Rapid increase in tumor size, involvement of surrounding tissues, and cortical destruction suggests malignancy, although they are not pathognomonic. Although clinicians often associate pain with

[a] Division of Thoracic Surgery, University of Toronto, Toronto General Hospital, 200 Elizabeth Street, 9N955, Toronto, ON M5G 2C4, Canada
[b] University Health Network, Toronto General Hospital, Toronto, ON, Canada
* Corresponding author. Division of Thoracic Surgery, University of Toronto, Toronto General Hospital, 200 Elizabeth Street, 9N955, Toronto, ON M5G 2C4, Canada.
E-mail address: Shaf.Keshavjee@uhn.on.ca

Thorac Surg Clin 20 (2010) 495–507
doi:10.1016/j.thorsurg.2010.07.003

Table 1
Classification of primary chest wall tumors

Bone Tumors	Benign	Malignant
Bone	Osteoblastoma Osteoid osteoma	Ewing sarcoma Osteosarcoma
Cartilage	Chondroma (enchondroma) Osteochondroma	Chondrosarcoma
Fibrous tissue	Fibrous dysplasia	
Bone marrow	Eosinophilic granuloma	Solitary plasmacytoma
Osteoclast	Aneurysmal bone cyst Giant cell tumor (osteoclastoma)	
Vascular	Hemangioma Cystic angiomatosis	Hemangiosarcoma
Other	Mesenchymal hamartoma	
Soft Tissue Tumors		
Adipose tissue	Lipoma Ossifying lipoma	Liposarcoma
Fibrous tissue	Fibroma (desmoid tumor) Ossifying fibroma	Fibrosarcoma MFH
Muscle	Leiomyoma Rhabdomyoma	Leiomyosarcoma Rhabdomyosarcoma Tendon sheath sarcoma
Nerve	Neurofibroma Schwannoma (neurilemmoma or neurinoma)	Askin tumor (PNET) Malignant schwannoma Neurofibrosarcoma Neuroblastoma
Vascular	Hemangioma Vascular leiomyoma	Hemangiosarcoma
Other		Hodgkin disease Leukemia Lymphoma Lymphosarcoma Mixed sarcoma Reticulosarcoma

malignant chest wall tumors, pain is not a reliable predictor of malignancy. Similarly, fixation to underlying tissues is not helpful in diagnosing malignant lesions, because it can be found in both malignant and benign conditions. There are no specific signs or symptoms that distinguish between benign and malignant lesions.[4]

Work-up should begin with a thorough history and physical examination. Imaging should be interpreted based on the location of the lesion and its size, the lesion's effect on the bone, the bone's response to the tumor, characteristics and composition of the tumor's matrix and cortex, and any evidence of a soft tissue mass.[5] Usually a chest radiograph is obtained first. Plain radiographs can demonstrate bony erosion of the lesion, lytic lesions, mediastinal lymphadenopathy or invasion, and the presence of any large pulmonary metastases. CT and MRI, however, are the critical imaging modalities. A chest CT assesses the extent of bone, soft tissue, pleural and mediastinal involvement, and pulmonary metastases and helps with surgical planning. It is more sensitive than plain films for determining bony cortical destruction or tumor matrix calcification.[6] MRI further delineates soft tissue, vascular and nerve involvement, and the presence of spinal cord or epidural extension, which is particularly helpful in delineating anatomic relationships of tumors in the thoracic inlet.[7] In general, benign bony lesions are small, with distinct geographic margins, whereas their malignant counterparts are permeative with bony destruction and show a sunburst pattern. Osteosarcomas and Ewing sarcomas may also demonstrate elevation of the periosteum at the interface of the tumor as it expands, referred to as Codman triangle.[8] Benign soft tissue tumors are often small and superficial, and certain tumors have classic appearances on imaging. Malignant tumors are often deep to the fascia and appear dark on T1-weighted MRI images and bright on T2-weighted MRI images. Radionucleotide bone scanning is done to rule out bony metastases.

Although imaging characteristics can suggest diagnosis of bony lesions, many soft tissue tumors require tissue for diagnosis. Biopsy methods include core needle as well as open incisional and excisional biopsy techniques. Although core needle may allow differentiation between benign and malignant processes, it may not provide sufficient tissue for histopathologic subtyping or genetic analysis. For lesions less than 2 cm, thought to be benign, and where primary closure is possible, excisional biopsy is recommended. If larger than 2 cm or suspicious for a primary malignancy, however, an incisional biopsy should be done. Incisional biopsies should measure a minimum of 1 cm^3 and be delivered fresh to pathology to allow diagnosis while allowing later complete wide excision. Care should be taken with the size and orientation of the biopsy because it must be completely incorporated in any future definitive surgical excision. The lesion should be approached directly to avoid contamination of unaffected structures. The creation of flaps or extensive dissection is contraindicated. For non-palpable lesions, preoperative wire localization or injection of methylene blue into the skin, soft tissue, and bone cortex can help localize the lesion.

LOCATION
Primary Tumors of the Rib

Primary tumors of the rib comprise only 5% to 7% of all primary bone neoplasms[9,10] but make up 50% of bony malignant tumors and the majority of benign bony tumors of the chest wall. Tumors of the rib are derived from bone, cartilage, bone marrow, vascular, or neural structures. Of the benign lesions, fibrous dysplasia and chondroma are the most common,[9] whereas chondrosarcoma and osteosarcoma are the most common malignant rib lesions.[11] Ewing sarcoma is the most common malignant rib tumor in the pediatric population.[10] The location within the rib can help with the diagnosis of the tumor. Chondromas and chondrosarcomas occur anteriorly at the costochondral junctions. PNET (Askin) tumors and hemangiopericytomas occur posteriorly on the chest wall adjacent to the vertebral column. In addition, size may help predict malignant potential. In a 13-year retrospective review at Children's Hospital Boston of all pediatric rib lesions that were evaluated and treated surgically, benign rib lesions were found significantly smaller, with a mean diameter of

3.2 cm, compared with malignant lesions, with a mean diameter of 7.2 cm.[10] Resection of malignant tumors should include wide resection of the rib with 4- to 5-cm proximal and distal margins, resection of portions of the ribs above and below the tumor, as well as adjacent muscles and underlying pleura and lung, if adherent.

Primary Tumors of the Clavicle and Scapula

Almost all bone lesions occurring in the skeleton can occur in the clavicle, but none is common. Up to 30% of malignant bony chest wall tumors originate in the scapula. Although uncommon, the benign soft tissue tumor classically found at the inferior angle of the scapula deep to the serratus anterior muscle is elastofibroma dorsi. Elastofibroma dorsi tumors typically occur in elderly women, are slow growing, and have a right-sided predominance, although up to 66% are bilateral.[12] Patients often present after developing symptoms, including pain and restriction of movement, and, although unclear, their pathogenesis may be related to repetitive movement or trauma. Typical MRI features include a sickle-shaped mass of generally low signal intensity with areas of high signal intensity on T1 and T2 images.[13] Complete surgical resection is recommended if the diagnosis is unclear or if the patients are symptomatic. Pathology reveals a nonencapsulated fibrous mass with streaks of fat within the tissue. There have been no reported incidents of malignant transformation of elastofibroma dorsi.[12]

Primary Tumors of the Sternum

Tumors of the sternum are usually malignant. Most common primary tumors of the sternum are osteosarcomas and chondrosarcomas.[1,14,15] In Chapelier and colleagues'[16] case series of 38 patients undergoing sternal resection and reconstruction for primary tumors, approximately 50% were found in previous irradiation fields. The size and location of the tumor determines the extent of resection. Upper-third lesions require resection of the manubrium and sternal body as well as resection of the medial ends of the clavicles and adjacent sternocostal cartilages (**Fig. 1**). Any involved adjacent structures, including lung, pericardium, or vessels, should be excised en bloc with the tumor. Middle-third lesions require resection of the sternal body, with preservation of the manubrium and xiphoid, if possible[4] (**Fig. 2**). Because these resections typically are extensive, they require planning for both skeletal and soft tissue reconstruction, often with composite prostheses, such as Marlex methyl methacrylate (**Fig. 3**). Soft tissue coverage to protect mediastinal structures

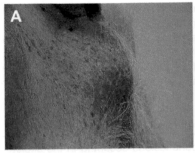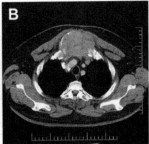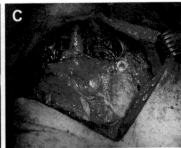

Fig. 1. (*A*) Visible anterior upper chest wall mass on physical examination; (*B*) CT chest demonstrating large soft tissue inhomogenous mass with central necrosis eroding manubrium and proximal sternal body; and (*C*) resection of mass including manubrium, proximal sternum, anterior first and second ribs, and medial ends of clavicles.

is obtained with muscle or myocutaneous flaps, with the pectoralis major muscle most frequently used.[15,16] Survival is related to sarcoma histologic type and grade.[17,18] Wide resection, with a minimum 3-cm margin, is necessary to reduce local recurrence in surrounding soft tissue.[16]

BONE TUMORS
Benign Bone Tumors

The most common benign bony tumors of the chest wall include fibrous dysplasia (30%–50%), osteochondroma (30%–50%), chondroma (10%–25%), aneurysmal bone cyst (10%–25%), and eosinophilic granuloma,[1] with many other rarer tumors reported in the literature (see **Table 1**).

Fibrous dysplasia
Fibrous dysplasia is a developmental skeletal disorder where normal bone marrow and cancellous bone is replaced by fibrous stroma and immature bone. Patients with fibrous dysplasia typically present with a painless mass in the posterior chest. Seventy to 80% of cases are monostotic, with only one bone involved.[6] Polyostotic fibrous dysplasia, where more than one bone is involved, is much less common in chest wall and rib lesions, although it can occur in the context of McCune-Albright syndrome, which is

associated with café au lait spots, and endocrine disorders, including Cushing syndrome, hyperthyroidism, and acromegaly as well as classically short stature and precocious puberty.[5] Fibrous dysplasia occurs most commonly in the second and third decades, with equal frequency in both genders. Pain develops if there is an associated pathologic fracture or as growth causes periosteal stretching. Its radiographic appearance is variable (**Fig. 4**). On chest radiograph it is seen as a rib deformity with a central fibrous area with fusiform expansion, a thin cortex, and often a lytic component. As it matures, this lesion often has a ground glass appearance due to variable degrees of ossification within the lesion causing an increase in its density. On CT, amorphous or irregular calcifications may be seen.[6] Histologically, the lesion consists of irregularly shaped spicules of bone, that have been termed *Chinese characters*, due to their shape, with fibrous stroma consisting of regular spindle cells.[19] Resection is only indicated for pain or if the diagnosis is in question.

Osteochondroma
Osteochondromas typically present in the second decade of life. They account for 50% of all benign bone tumors, with the rib, particularly at the costochondral junction, the most common location.

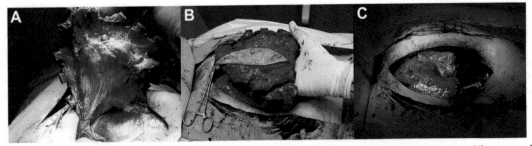

Fig. 2. (*A*) Sarcoma of the middle third of the sternum, with complete resection of the sternum; (*B*) extent of surgical resection, including soft tissue and skin; and (*C*) size of defect after resection.

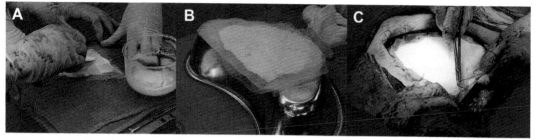

Fig. 3. Creation of methyl methacrylate mesh sandwich. (*A*) Methyl methacrylate paste is first applied between two layers of polypropylene mesh; (*B*) the methyl methacrylate mesh sandwich prosthesis is dried after conforming it to the shape of the defect; and (*C*) the mesh is sutured in with polypropylene sutures to cover the bony defect of a sternal body resection. No muscle or skin flap was required.

They account for only 2.7% to 8.5% of primary rib tumors.[9] Most are round and measure less than 9 cm. Imaging is usually adequate for diagnosis, demonstrating punctate or flocculent calcifications with a mineralized hyaline cartilage cap best seen on CT. The cortex and medullary space blend into the underlying bone, which is how a definitive diagnosis is made on CT or MRI.[6] These tumors can be observed with serial imaging. Cartilage caps thicker than 2 cm in adults and 3 cm in children, however, are suspicious for malignant degeneration to chondrosarcoma or osteosarcoma and should be treated aggressively with wide local excision.

Chondroma
Also referred to as enchondromas, chondromas are benign cartilaginous tumors originating from the medullary cavity. They represent 2.8% to 12.2% of all primary rib tumors[9] and are typically

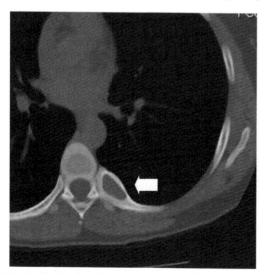

Fig. 4. Fibrous dysplasia of posterior eighth rib seen as a solitary, lytic expansile lesion on CT chest (*arrow*). There is no evidence of any overlying periosteal reaction, cortical disruption or soft tissue reaction around the lesion.

found in the anterior portion of the rib. Plain film radiographs demonstrate a slow-growing, well-demarcated, osteolytic lesion with mild expansion and well-defined sclerotic margins. Punctate calcifications of the matrix and scalloping of the cortex are often seen, especially on CT and MRI.[9] Microscopically, they have nodules of hyaline cartilage with chondrocytes containing small, condensed nuclei. Chondromas can be difficult to differentiate from low-grade chondrosarcomas, even microscopically, and should, therefore, all be treated with wide local excision.

Langerhans cell histiocytosis/eosinophilic granuloma
Characterized by idiopathic proliferation of histiocytes, eosinophilic granuloma is one of the syndromes seen with Langerhans cell histiocytosis that produce single or multiple expanding erosive bony lesions. Langerhans cell histiocytosis rarely arises from the chest wall but has been reported in the ribs and sternum. A multifocal multisystem disease, Langerhans cell histiocytosis in the bones is characterized by focal lytic lesions with or without bone expansion and destruction. Diagnosis is made with core needle or open biopsy by identifying Birbeck granules on electron microscopy. Rib lesions account for approximately 10% of solitary eosinophilic granuloma,[20] and are more commonly found in adults. Patients with Langerhans cell histiocytosis typically present with systemic symptoms of fever and leukocytosis in association with localized pain. The lesions are generally osteolytic on imaging, with no matrix mineralization, which makes them radiolucent. Treatment includes intralesional and systemic steroids, systemic chemotherapy,[7] and low-dose radiotherapy for residual disease or high-grade tumors. Surgical resection is not indicated.

Aneurysmal bone cyst
Aneurysmal bone cysts are rare, benign, locally aggressive expansile cystic osteolytic lesions,

accounting for approximately 5% of all primary rib lesions.[21] Their underlying cause is uncertain, although possibly originating as arteriovenous malformations. These tumors may also be associated with cystic changes in angiomas, chondroblastomas, fibrous dysplasia, giant cell tumors, and osteoblastomas and can coexist with these lesions. The majority (75%) present before 20 years of age. Aneurysmal bone cysts most commonly involve the posterior elements of the spine in the chest wall as well as the posterior or lateral aspects of any of the ribs.[9] Radiographs demonstrate a well-defined expansile lytic lesion. In early stages, they are confined to the cortex but can progress to erode through the medullary portion of the bone, with soft tissue extension, making them difficult to differentiate from sarcomas. MRI may show fluid-fluid levels within multiseptated hemorrhagic cysts in the tumor, but these fluid levels can also be seen with simple bone cysts, giant cell tumors, and chondroblastomas.[6] Microscopically, these tumors have blood-filled spaces without endothelial cell linings. Open biopsy is often needed to obtain diagnosis because needle biopsies usually only get a return of blood. Complete excision is recommended for symptomatic lesions.

Osteoid osteoma

Osteoid osteomas are benign osteoblastic tumors. They typically present in the first two decades of life. Most occur in the posterior elements of the spine. Only 0.23% to 2% occur in ribs, and osteoid osteoma accounts for only 1% to 1.4% of primary rib tumors. They occur in the posterior portion of the rib and may lead to scoliosis. The most defining symptom of osteoid osteoma is night pain that responds to both nonsteroidal anti-inflammatories and salicylates. Imaging reveals a small (<1 cm) radiolucent lesion, termed a *nidus*, best seen on CT, with a thick sclerotic margin of reactive bone.[1] These tumors have increased uptake on bone scintigraphy and show soft tissue edema on MRI. Pathologically, the nidus contains osteoids at its center, with maturation into bone trabeculae in a fibrovascular stroma. Treatment is generally with radiofrequency ablation, and resection is rarely required.

Osteoblastoma

Osteoblastomas, rare benign osteoblastic tumors, thought to be on continuum of osteoid osteomas, typically affect the posterior and posterolateral shaft of the rib. Imaging reveals a well-defined osteolytic lesion (>2 cm) with slight expansion but with a sharp sclerotic rim. CT allows accurate delineation of osseous involvement and type of calcification. These tumors demonstrate increased uptake on bone scans. Histologically, osteoblastomas are characterized by interconnected trabeculae of bone in a fibrovascular stroma.[5]

Giant cell tumor

Giant cell tumors, benign lesions, are common. They present between the ages of 20 and 40 years, more frequently in men than women. Consisting of vascular sinuses lined and filled with giant cells and spindle cells, radiographs demonstrate eccentric, osteolytic expansile masses with cortical thinning. Giant cell tumors often present with a soft tissue mass. CT helps define the extent of tumor involvement of surrounding structures. MRI is better with soft tissue delineation, in which giant cell tumors are dark on both T1- and T2-weighted images. Although generally considered benign, these tumors are locally aggressive and have a 30% to 50% risk of local recurrence[9] and may even rarely metastasize.[5]

Malignant Bone Tumors

In descending order of incidence, chondrosarcoma, Ewing sarcoma, osteosarcoma, and solitary plasmacytoma are the most common malignant bony tumors of the chest wall. Although multiple myeloma, presenting as a solitary plamacytoma, often appears in the literature as the most common malignancy of the bony chest wall, it is more accurately defined as a local presentation of a systemic disease and not a primary chest wall lesion.[1] The rib is the most common bone involved in malignant tumors of the chest wall, followed by the scapula, sternum, and clavicle.

Chondrosarcoma

Chondrosarcoma is the most common primary bone tumor of the chest wall in adults.[22] Originating from cartilage, chondrosarcomas may develop de novo from normal bone or can degenerate from benign cartilage tumors, such as chondromas, exostoses, or osteochondromas. They are, therefore, typically found anteriorly in the chest wall or in the sternum. On imaging, they demonstrate bony destruction, irregular contours, and varying degrees of calcification.[23] Early-stage lesions demonstrate a thickened cortex whereas higher-grade lesions usually have complete cortical destruction, along with a soft tissue mass (**Fig. 5**). Alternatively, the growth of a benign cartilage tumor or expansion of their cartilage cap may suggest malignant degeneration. CT and MRI allow determination of tumor extension as well as areas of scattered calcification in the chondroid matrix.[24] Pathologically, the tumor demonstrates a chondroid matrix with increased cellularity, binucleate cells,

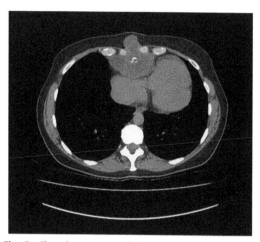

Fig. 5. Chondrosarcoma of the sternum with cortical destruction, soft tissue extension posteriorly into the mediastinum and anteriorly into subcutaneous tissues, focal calcification within the tumor, and compression of both the right ventricle and atrium, as seen on CT chest.

with the degree of cellularity, mitoses, and cytologic atypia determining tumor grade. These tumors are unresponsive to chemotherapy or radiation and, therefore, complete wide local surgical resection is the only chance of cure.

Ewing sarcoma

Malignant, small, round cell–type tumors are a highly malignant group of tumors that share a common (t11;22) (q24;q12) translocation.[25] They include Ewing sarcoma and PNETs, also known as Askin tumors. Typically occurring in children to young adults, with a male predominance of 1.6:1,[24] 6.5% of malignant small round cell–type tumors arise in the chest wall, with a single rib the most common site of occurrence,[3] followed by the clavicle, then scapula. Approximately 15% of Ewing sarcomas[24] and 50% of PNETs arise in the chest wall.[26] Malignant small round cell–type tumors often present with a painful chest wall mass associated with systemic symptoms, such as fever, malaise, and weight loss. Dyspnea, caused by associated pleural or pericardial effusions, is also common. Imaging demonstrates a large, noncalcified, soft tissue mass associated with bone destruction. The periosteal reaction classically takes on an onion peel or sunburst appearance. Diagnosis is made with incisional biopsy, with demonstration of small round blue cells with scanty clear cytoplasm and positive staining on periodic acid–Schiff due to the presence of glycogen. Rosettes, dark oval nuclei with neurofibrillary cores, are found in PNETs and not in Ewing, and are, therefore, used to distinguish

between the two tumors.[27] Treatment is neoadjuvant chemotherapy, followed by surgical resection if the tumor is well demarcated, and can be completely resected with wide resection. Chemotherapy often shrinks the tumor, making subsequent chest wall resection less morbid as well as increasing overall 5-year survival to approximately 60%.[28] Resection, however, should incorporate the pretreatment extent of disease. Radiotherapy is less frequently used today as postoperative adjuvant treatment. The addition of myeloablative therapy and stem cell rescue may improve outcome in patients with primary metastatic Ewing sarcoma.[29] Bilateral whole-lung radiation may improve event-free survival in patients with lung, bone, or bone marrow metastases.[3]

Osteosarcoma

Osteosarcoma is the most common overall bone tumor, but in chest wall bony tumors it is second after chondrosarcomas. Osteosarcomas generally present in puberty. In a recent review of the literature by Eyre and colleagues,[30] consisting of small number of case-control and cohort studies, possible risk factors for the development of osteosarcoma emerged. These included environmental triggers, such as high fluoride exposure and residency on a farm or a parent working as a farmer, as well as genetic predisposition: family history of malignancy, younger age at puberty, association with other musculoskeletal anomalies, and multiple birth defects. Retinoblastoma (RB1 mutation on chromosome 13q14) carries a 500× to 1000× risk of developing osteosarcoma than the general population and Li-Fraumeni syndrome (p53 mutation) a 15-fold increased risk. Osteosarcomas typically arise from a rib, scapula, or clavicle. On CT and MRI they are osteoblastic lesions that demonstrate bone destruction with a large heterogeneous mass due to hemorrhage or necrosis. They demonstrate a pattern of mineralization concentrated at the center of the lesion (**Fig. 6**).[23] On biopsy these tumor cells are spindle-shaped, epithelioid, or small and round, with osteoid matrix calcification. Unlike chondrosarcomas, these tumors are responsive to chemotherapy and are treated first with neoadjuvant chemotherapy followed by surgery.[24,31] In the event of metastases, subsequent pulmonary metastectomy can increase long-term disease-free survival and overall survival. Even with adjuvant treatment, however, the overall 5-year survival for osteosarcoma has been reported as low as 15%.[4]

Solitary plasmacytoma

Solitary plasmacytomas are uncommon solitary lesions, which, unlike disseminated myeloma, are treated with surgical resection or with local

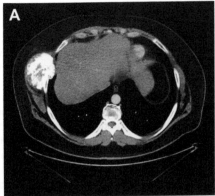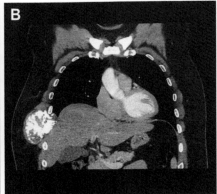

Fig. 6. (*A*) Axial and (*B*) coronal CT chest images of an osteosarcoma of the right chest wall at the level of sixth rib with rib involvement and extension into subcutaneous tissue.

irradiation. Two-thirds of patients progress to develop generalized myeloma within 3 years of diagnosis, with poor prognosis, but the remainder of the patients achieve permanent cure.

BENIGN SOFT TISSUE TUMORS

The differential of soft tissue abnormalities is vast and, in addition to primary tumors, should encompass local presentations of systemic diseases as well as infectious causes, such as tuberculosis and actinomycosis. In terms of primary benign soft tissue tumors (see **Table 1**), the most common diagnoses include lipomas, fibromas, hemangiomas, and giant cell tumors.[32] Less common diagnoses include lipoblastomas and mesenchymal hamartomas.

Lipomas

Lipomas are well-circumscribed adipose masses that can occur in patients of any age but are typically found in obese and older patients between the ages of 50 and 70 years of age. On the chest wall, they are often larger and deeper than lipomas on other sites of the body. CT and MRI demonstrate homogenous masses consistent with mature fatty tissue. They can be difficult to differentiate from low-grade liposarcomas on imaging.

Lipoblastoma

Lipoblastomas are uncommon benign tumors of fetal embryonic fat that present as a painless chest wall mass in infants. These tumors are bright on T1-weighted MRI, and, although benign, they often have intercostal extensions. Wide local resection is, therefore, required to ensure negative margins.

Fibromas and Fibromatosis

Fibromas are localized benign tumors of connective tissue, also termed *desmoid tumors*. Although considered benign, these tumors can be locally aggressive. They are seen in association with Gardner syndrome (mutation of the adenomatous polyposis coli gene) and in scars of previous thoracotomies.[7] Surgical resection with negative margins is required to prevent local recurrence, because they have local recurrence rates up to 70%.[4,33] Aggressive fibromatosis describes a more extensive infiltrative disease of fibrous scar tissue. It is treated with either wide excision or, if unresectable, chemotherapy and radiation.[20]

Hemangiomas

Hemangiomas are usually large, benign proliferations of blood vessels that form within subcutaneous tissue, muscle, ribs, or vertebrae. They usually occur before the age of 30 and are uncommon on the chest wall. CT demonstrates heterogeneous soft tissue masses with fatty, fibrous, and vascular elements. Ultrasound can be used to determine flow within the lesion and MRI to show vascular and adipose components of the lesion. In infants, cavernous hemangiomata can cause fetal hydrops and death due to cardiac failure from arteriovenous malformation and shunting. Thrombocytopenia is also seen in Kasabach-Merritt syndrome due to platelet sequestration.[26]

Benign Peripheral Nerve Sheath Tumors

Benign peripheral nerve sheath tumors consist of neurofibromas and schwannomas, also referred to as neurilemmomas and neurinomas. Schwannomas are encapsulated tumors that originate from intercostal nerves or spinal nerve roots. They are usually only seen on CT or MRI as a homogenous mass, although bone scalloping may be seen on plain radiographs. They are extremely painful on biopsy, giving a diagnostic clue as to their origin. Neurofibromas originate from peripheral nerves and in up to 60% can be associated with neurofibromatosis type I, multiple plexiform neurofibromas, or multiple endocrine neoplasia.[26] They are slow-growing masses, often occurring between the ages of 20 and 30 years.[6] They may demonstrate cystic degeneration, with a central zone that is more cellular and a peripheral more stromal zone, creating a target appearance on both T2-weighted images and gadolinium-enhanced MRI. These tumors can grow into the spinal canal in a dumbbell fashion.

Mesenchymal Hamartomas

Mesenchymal hamartomas, also referred to as mesenchymomas, present in infancy, often with chest deformity and respiratory distress. These large tumors can be solitary or multifocal and must be differentiated from aneurysmal bone cysts and chondromas. Partially calcified on imaging, they often demonstrate chondroid tissue mixed with immature mesenchyme, osteoclasts, and endothelium-lined blood spaces on pathology. Wide local excision is recommended if there is respiratory or cardiac compromise.[7]

MALIGNANT SOFT TISSUE TUMORS

More common than malignant tumors of the bony thorax, most malignant soft tissue tumors of the chest wall are sarcomas, including malignant fibrous histiocytomas, liposarcomas, and fibrosarcomas. They are often asymptomatic and more commonly found on the anterior chest wall. Most sarcomas have a poor prognosis, with survival influenced by histology, tumor grade, diameter, and location. Reported overall 5-year survival is still only 50% to 66%, although low-grade well-differentiated tumors treated with wide local excision can achieve 5-year survival rates up to 90%.[34] The mnemonic, SCARE, is used to recall those sarcomas that most commonly metastasize to lymph nodes: synovial sarcoma, clear cell, angiosarcoma, rhabdomyosarcoma, and epithelioid sarcoma.[35]

Malignant Fibrous Histiocytoma

Malignant fibrous histiocytoma usually occurs in older patients but has a bimodal distribution, with a first peak from 20 to 30 years of age, and a second, larger peak from ages 50 to 60. Although they are the most common radiation-induced tumor[24] and the most common soft-tissue tumor in adults, they rarely arise from the chest wall. On imaging, they are heterogeneous with ill-defined contours. MFH is generally diagnosed with biopsy and treated with neoadjuvant chemotherapy, followed by surgical resection and further adjuvant chemotherapy.[24]

Synovial Sarcomas

Synovial sarcomas are extremely rare in the chest wall. Presenting in adolescence to early adulthood, they are calcified in 20% to 30% of patients. These heterogeneous masses demonstrate fluid-fluid levels on MRI due to hemorrhage and necrosis within their cystic components. Treatment includes excision followed by adjuvant radiation, although radiation can also be used preoperatively. These tumors can also be treated with chemotherapy, because they are 50% chemosensitive.[36] Five-year survival is approximately 50%.[24]

Rhabdomyosarcoma

Uncommon in adults, rhabdomyosarcoma is the second most common malignant chest wall tumor in children. These tumors are treated with neoadjuvant chemotherapy and radiotherapy, followed by surgical resection, then ongoing chemotherapy and radiation.[28] Negative prognostic features include alveolar subtype (compared with embryonal subtype), invasive tumors greater than 10 cm, and R1 resections.[28] Preoperative work-up should include MRI of the primary tumor and full staging with CT thorax, abdominal ultrasound, and bone scans to rule out metastatic disease. These are aggressive tumors and only approximately 10% of rhabdomyosarcomas are resectable.[26]

Fibrosarcoma

Fibrosarcomas occur in adults as heterogeneous masses on CT and MRI, due to necrosis and hemorrhage. Treatment includes neoadjuvant chemotherapy followed by resection. Postoperative radiation is used for positive margins. These lesions tend to both recur locally and metastasize. Neurofibrosarcomas typically present with an enlarging painful mass. Also referred to as malignant schwannomas or malignant peripheral nerve sheath tumors, neurofibrosarcomas often originate from neurofibromas of spinal nerve roots or intercostal nerves or in the brachial plexus. They are most common in adults and can be associated with previous irradiation. Close to one-third (29%) of patients with neurofibromatosis develop neurofibrosarcomas.[24]

Other Primary Malignant Tumors

Many other sarcomas, including leiomyosarcomas and neuroblastomas, can arise infrequently in the chest wall. Leiomyosarcomas, arising from blood vessels, including pulmonary arteries, can also present in cutaneous and subcutaneous tissues. Arising in adulthood, they have been associated with immunosuppression, including organ transplantation, AIDS, and Epstein-Barr virus. They are painful and unresponsive to chemotherapy. Neuroblastomas uncommonly involve the chest wall primarily. They arise in sympathetic nervous tissue, usually before the age of 5. They can invade the neural foramina causing a dumbbell appearance. Localized excision is the treatment of choice, possibly followed by boost of external beam radiation.[7]

Undifferentiated or spindle cell sarcomas are those sarcomas that cannot be more accurately classified. These sarcomas are often large, with heterogeneous attenuation and signal intensity on CT and MRI, respectively. Treatment typically involves resection and radiation, with the addition of chemotherapy preoperatively in some cases to shrink tumors initially judged unresectable.

Systemic Diseases

Although not considered primary lesions of the chest wall, systemic diseases can present as chest wall masses that can be confused with chest wall tumors and, therefore, are briefly discussed. Both leukemia and lymphoma can present as a chest wall mass. Multiple bone lesions are often seen with leukemia. Lymphoma can present as primary bone lymphoma, multifocal lymphoma, or lymphoma with both nodal and osseous disease.[26] Diagnosis is made with a biopsy. Classically, Reed-Sternberg cells are seen in Hodgkin lymphoma, and flow cytometry or immunohistochemistry is used to determine cell lineage in non-Hodgkin lymphoma. Treatment is systemic chemotherapy. Surgical resection is not generally indicated.[7]

Myeloma, a malignant tumor of plasma cells, accounts for 50% of malignant bony tumors of the chest wall but is not considered a primary tumor. It is associated with multiple bone sites with widespread osteolytic bone destruction, hypercalcemia, renal dysfunction, and refractory anemia. A solitary lesion associated with multiple myeloma is termed a solitary plasmacytoma (discussed previously). Diagnosis is made with monoclonal elevation of IgG, IgA, or Bence Jones light chains on serum immune electrophoresis. Chemotherapy, with autogenous bone marrow transplantation, is commonly used as standard treatment,

with radiation for localized areas of symptomatic involvement. In the chest wall, surgical resection is not indicated.

Infections can also present as a chest wall mass or abscess, either as a primary site or as local extension from a deep chest infection (ie, empyema or mediastinitis). A diagnosis of tuberculosis is aided by a positive contact or travel history, in combination with mediastinal lymphadenopathy. Surgical drainage and resection, with débridement of any necrotic bone or tissue, is the treatment of choice in combination with systemic antituberculous treatment. Actinomycosis can also mimic a chest wall tumor with rib destruction. It is diagnosed by the development of sinus tracts and pathognomonic sulfur granules on fine needle aspiration. Treatment is with systemic penicillin G, with possible surgical drainage or resection if required.[7]

SURGICAL TREATMENT OF CHEST WALL TUMORS

The indication for surgery is based on evaluation of the tumor histology, location, degree of local invasion, and presence of metastases. Localization of small tumors, or for those with significant response to neoadjuvant treatment, may be difficult. Video-assisted thoracoscopic surgery may facilitate tumor localization if the tumor is visible from the pleural surface. Entering the pleura one or two ribs above or below the lesion may allow palpation of the defect. If the lesion is too small to be observed directly or by palpation, preoperative coil wire placement by interventional radiology or the use of image-guided methylene blue injection into surrounding tissues allows intraoperative localization and resection.

Most chest wall tumors are treated primarily with surgical resection. Exceptions include Ewing sarcoma and solitary plasmacytomas. Ewing sarcoma is first treated with sequential chemotherapy and radiation, followed by possible surgical resection. Solitary plasmacytoma is treated solely with radiation. Surgical resection of all tumors must ensure negative margins to prevent local recurrence, although the exact margin size is somewhat debated depending on the specific tumor type. Most benign tumors are excised with simply negative margins, whereas many agree that locally aggressive benign lesions and malignant tumors require a minimum 4 cm margin for wide excision. With rib lesions, the excision should generally incorporate resection of all or most of the rib involved, a portion of any adjacent ribs, and en bloc resection of any attached structures, including portions of pleura, lung, pericardium, thymus, or diaphragm. Malignant tumors of the manubrium, sternum, clavicle, and scapula generally require excision of the entire bone and surrounding soft tissue to ensure negative margins.

Reconstruction

Chest wall surgery must be carefully planned to ensure accurate localization of the lesion, complete resection, and adequate tissue coverage, with minimum morbidity. Chest wall closure for smaller lesions can usually be done primarily, but for larger tumors in which a considerable defect is anticipated, both skeletal reconstruction and soft tissue coverage are often necessary. Involvement of a multidisciplinary team, including plastic surgeons, is often invaluable. Although there is no true consensus, in general, chest wall defects are reconstructed when they measure more than 10 cm posteriorly, greater than 5 cm in any other location, or are located where the scapular tip falls (to prevent a trapped scapula). Subscapular and apical chest wall resections generally do not require reconstruction. In a report of 500 chest wall reconstructions, 275 of which were performed for chest wall tumors, the majority underwent pedicled or myocutaneous flaps with pectoralis major or latissimus dorsi, although serratus anterior, rectus abdominis, and external oblique muscles were also used. Synthetic materials used included polypropylene (Marlex) or polytetrafluoroethylene mesh.[37] Others report use of omental, thoracoepigastric fasciocutaneous, and chimeric flaps as well as reconstruction with methyl methacrylate sandwiched between two layers of polypropylene mesh to provide chest wall stability, protect underlying vital structures, and restore body contour (see **Fig. 3**).[38] Choice of reconstruction depends somewhat on the expertise and preferences of the involved thoracic and reconstructive surgeons. In general, latissimus dorsi flaps are used for large posterior defects and pectoralis major flaps for anterior defects.

Postoperative respiratory morbidity is related to impaired respiratory function and chest mechanics after chest wall resection. Complications have been reported in 46% to 69% of patients,[39,40] with respiratory complications in up to 24%,[41] often due to a flail segment created resulting in paradoxic movement, atelectasis, pooling of secretions, and subsequent respiratory failure, pneumonia, or acute respiratory distress syndrome. For large defects, it is thus desirable to use the Marlex methyl methacrylate composite reconstruction technique to provide a chest wall reconstruction with stability to prevent flail and respiratory compromise. Other common complications include wound infections and cardiac arrhythmias. In a recent series of 262 chest wall resections, in which 251 were for tumors, significant predictors of postoperative complications were patient age, concomitant anatomic lung parenchymal resection, and increased size of chest wall defect resected.[41] Risk factors for wound infection include tumor ulceration and the use of omentum in soft tissue reconstruction.[42]

Adjuvant Treatment

Multimodality therapy is critical in the treatment of specific chest wall tumors. The use of multiagent chemotherapy both in the neoadjuvant and adjuvant settings for osteosarcoma and malignant small round cell–type tumors (Ewing sarcoma and PNETs) has been critical in significantly improving the overall and disease-free survival of patients with these tumors. The use of adjuvant radiotherapy is also used with certain tumors, including malignant soft tissue tumors and osteosarcomas, to prevent local recurrence and to treat recurrent tumors.

SUMMARY

The differential diagnosis of patients presenting with a lesion on the chest wall must take into account local anatomy as well as patient age, gender, previous history of malignancy, and exposure to radiation. In addition to benign or malignant primary chest wall tumors, diagnostic possibilities include local presentations of systemic disease, infection, metastasis, or extension of underlying malignancies. With particular attention to imaging characteristics of the lesion, a diagnosis can often be made. Use of plain radiographs, CT, and MRI further facilitate decision making in how to best obtain tissue diagnosis without compromising potential future surgical resection and allows for operative planning. Treatment decisions are guided by the local aggressiveness of the tumor, its malignant potential, and its responsiveness to chemotherapy and radiotherapy. These tumors should be assessed and treated in a multidisciplinary setting, with a priori involvement of thoracic surgery, medical, and radiation oncology as well as plastic surgery when reconstruction is required, so that an appropriately ordered multimodality treatment plan can be set in place to optimize patient outcome.

REFERENCES

1. Faber LP, Somers J, Templeton AC. Chest wall tumors. Curr Probl Surg 1995;32(8):661–747.

2. Hsu PK, Hsu HS, Lee HC, et al. Management of primary chest wall tumors: 14 years' clinical experience. J Chin Med Assoc 2006;69(8):377–82.

3. Dang NC, Siegel SE, Phillips JD. Malignant chest wall tumors in children and young adults. J Pediatr Surg 1999;34(12):1773–8.

4. Athanassiadi K, Kalavrouziotis G, Rondogianni D, et al. Primary chest wall tumors: early and long-term results of surgical treatment. Eur J Cardiothorac Surg 2001;19(5):589–93.

5. Levesque J, Marx R, Bell RS, et al. A clinical guide to primary bone tumors. Baltimore (MD): Williams & Williams; 1998.

6. Tateishi U, Gladish GW, Kusumoto M, et al. Chest wall tumors: radiologic findings and pathologic correlation: part 1. Benign tumors. Radiographics 2003;23(6):1477–90.

7. La Quaglia MP. Chest wall tumors in childhood and adolescence. Semin Pediatr Surg 2008;17(3): 173–80.

8. Visotsky JL, Benson LS. Eponyms in orthopaedics. J Bone Joint Surg Am 2001;83(Suppl 2 Pt 2):123–7.

9. Hughes EK, James SL, Butt S, et al. Benign primary tumours of the ribs. Clin Radiol 2006;61(4):314–22.

10. Kim S, Lee S, Arsenault DA, et al. Pediatric rib lesions: a 13-year experience. J Pediatr Surg 2008; 43(10):1781–5.

11. Aydogdu K, Findik G, Agackiran Y, et al. Primary tumors of the ribs; experience with 78 patients. Interact Cardiovasc Thorac Surg 2009;9(2):251–4.

12. Mortman KD, Hochheiser GM, Giblin EM, et al. Elastofibroma dorsi: clinicopathologic review of 6 cases. Ann Thorac Surg 2007;83(5):1894–7.

13. Schafmayer C, Kahlke V, Leuschner I, et al. Elastofibroma dorsi as differential diagnosis in tumors of the thoracic wall. Ann Thorac Surg 2006;82(4): 1501–4.

14. Chapelier A, Macchiarini P, Rietjens M, et al. Chest wall reconstruction following resection of large primary malignant tumors. Eur J Cardiothorac Surg 1994;8(7):351–6 [discussion: 357].

15. Soysal O, Walsh GL, Nesbitt JC, et al. Resection of sternal tumors: extent, reconstruction, and survival. Ann Thorac Surg 1995;60(5):1353–8 [discussion: 1358–9].

16. Chapelier AR, Missana MC, Couturaud B, et al. Sternal resection and reconstruction for primary malignant tumors. Ann Thorac Surg 2004;77(3): 1001–6 [discussion: 1006–7].

17. King RM, Pairolero PC, Trastek VF, et al. Primary chest wall tumors: factors affecting survival. Ann Thorac Surg 1986;41(6):597–601.

18. Martini N, Huvos AG, Burt ME, et al. Predictors of survival in malignant tumors of the sternum. J Thorac Cardiovasc Surg 1996;111(1):96–105 [discussion: 105–6].

19. Vanderelst A, Spiegl G, de Francquen P. Fibrous dysplasia of the rib. J Belge Radiol 1988;71(6):742–3.

20. van den Berg H, van Rijn RR, Merks JH. Management of tumors of the chest wall in childhood: a review. J Pediatr Hematol Oncol 2008;30(3): 214–21.

21. Sadighi A, Tuccimei U, Annessi P. Aneurysmal bone cyst of the rib: a case report. Chir Ital 2006;58(3): 403–6.

22. Liptay MJ, Fry WA. Malignant bone tumors of the chest wall. Semin Thorac Cardiovasc Surg 1999; 11(3):278–84.

23. Tateishi U, Gladish GW, Kusumoto M, et al. Chest wall tumors: radiologic findings and pathologic correlation: part 2. Malignant tumors. Radiographics 2003;23(6):1491–508.

24. Gladish GW, Sabloff BM, Munden RF, et al. Primary thoracic sarcomas. Radiographics 2002;22(3): 621–37.

25. Kennedy JG, Frelinghuysen P, Hoang BH. Ewing sarcoma: current concepts in diagnosis and treatment. Curr Opin Pediatr 2003;15(1):53–7.

26. Watt AJ. Chest wall lesions. Paediatr Respir Rev 2002;3(4):328–38.

27. Wu JM, Montgomery E. Classification and pathology. Surg Clin North Am 2008;88(3):483–520, v–vi.

28. Saenz NC, Hass DJ, Meyers P, et al. Pediatric chest wall Ewing's sarcoma. J Pediatr Surg Apr 2000;35(4):550–5.

29. Paulussen M, Frohlich B, Jurgens H. Ewing tumour: incidence, prognosis and treatment options. Paediatr Drugs 2001;3(12):899–913.

30. Eyre R, Feltbower RG, Mubwandarikwa E, et al. Epidemiology of bone tumours in children and young adults. Pediatr Blood Cancer 2009;53(6): 941–52.

31. Bielack SS, Carrle D, Hardes J, et al. Bone tumors in adolescents and young adults. Curr Treat Options Oncol 2008;9(1):67–80.

32. Faber KJ, Patterson SD, Heathcote JG, et al. Osteoblastoma of the clavicle. J South Orthop Assoc 2003;12(2):66–70.

33. Abbas AE, Deschamps C, Cassivi SD, et al. Chestwall desmoid tumors: results of surgical intervention. Ann Thorac Surg 2004;78(4):1219–23 [discussion: 1219–23].

34. Gordon MS, Hajdu SI, Bains MS, et al. Soft tissue sarcomas of the chest wall. Results of surgical resection. J Thorac Cardiovasc Surg 1991;101(5): 843–54.

35. Riad S, Griffin AM, Liberman B, et al. Lymph node metastasis in soft tissue sarcoma in an extremity. Clin Orthop Relat Res 2004;426:129–34.

36. Hung JJ, Chou TY, Sun CH, et al. Primary synovial sarcoma of the posterior chest wall. Ann Thorac Surg 2008;85(6):2120–2.

37. Arnold PG, Pairolero PC. Chest-wall reconstruction: an account of 500 consecutive patients. Plast Reconstr Surg 1996;98(5):804–10.

38. Skoracki RJ, Chang DW. Reconstruction of the chest wall and thorax. J Surg Oncol 2006;94(6):455–65.

39. Mansour KA, Thourani VH, Losken A, et al. Chest wall resections and reconstruction: a 25-year experience. Ann Thorac Surg Jun 2002;73(6):1720–5 [discussion: 1725–6].

40. Deschamps C, Tirnaksiz BM, Darbandi R, et al. Early and long-term results of prosthetic chest wall reconstruction. J Thorac Cardiovasc Surg 1999; 117(3):588–91 [discussion: 591–2].

41. Weyant MJ, Bains MS, Venkatraman E, et al. Results of chest wall resection and reconstruction with and without rigid prosthesis. Ann Thorac Surg 2006;81(1):279–85.

42. Lans TE, van der Pol C, Wouters MW, et al. Complications in wound healing after chest wall resection in cancer patients; a multivariate analysis of 220 patients. J Thorac Oncol 2009;4(5): 639–43.

Surgery of the Chest Wall for Involvement by Breast Cancer

Massimiliano D'Aiuto, MD[a], Marcellino Cicalese, MD[b],
Giuseppe D'Aiuto, MD[a],
Gaetano Rocco, MD, FRCSEd, FETCS, FCCP[a,b],*

KEYWORDS

• Breast cancer • Chest wall • Surgery

Breast cancer is the most common tumor among women and is the second leading cause of cancer deaths, in women, after lung cancer.[1] According to the American Cancer Society, about 1.3 million women are diagnosed with breast cancer annually worldwide and about 465,000 die from the disease.[2] The overall survival (OS) is strongly influenced by the stage of the disease at the time of the diagnosis. According to the SEER (Surveillance Epidemiology and End Results) Summary Stage system, the 5-year relative breast cancer survival rate is 98% for localized disease, 84% for regional disease, and 23% for advanced disease.[3,4] Surgical management of localized primary tumor includes breast-conserving surgery plus radiation treatment (breast conservative therapy [BCT]), mastectomy plus reconstruction, and mastectomy alone. Sentinel lymph node (SLN) biopsy is the gold standard procedure to stage the node status and preludes to a complete axillary dissection when the SLN is involved.[5–9] Rarely, breast cancer may involve the chest wall structures at the time of the primary diagnosis. More frequently, chest wall infiltration occurs later in the event of locoregional relapse with or without concomitant metastatic disease. In both cases, surgical resection of the chest wall may be indicated as part of a multimodality treatment that should also include chemotherapy, radiotherapy, and the hormonal and biologic therapies. The main goal of chest wall resection (CWR) is the control of locoregional disease. However, even in the patient with metastatic disease, the CWR may provide good palliation and better quality of life.

CLINICAL FEATURE

Chest wall involvement by breast cancer most commonly presents as single or multiple, painless nodules and/or masses eventually infiltrating or ulcerating the overlying skin. Erythema or skin thickening, induration, widespread nodularity, and pruritic or nonpruritic papules may also be found. With advanced disease, the tumor may extend beyond the chest wall, determining the feature of carcinoma en cuirass. Signs of axillary disease may include a mobile mass into the axilla, arm edema, brachial plexopathy, pain, and decreased range of motion. Supraclavicular nodal disease most commonly presents as a painless mass detected during a routine physical examination. The presence of Rotter (interpectoral) nodes disease is revealed by submuscular mass palpable deep to the pectoralis major. The involvement of the internal mammary chain by breast cancer is often asymptomatic, although a painless subcutaneous parasternal mass with or without skin involvement may be observed as the disease progresses.

This work was not been supported and the authors have nothing to disclose.
[a] Department of Breast Surgery and Oncology, Division of Breast Surgery, National Cancer Institute, Pascale Foundation, Naples, Italy
[b] Department of Thoracic Surgery and Oncology, Division of Thoracic Surgery, National Cancer Institute, Pascale Foundation, Naples, Italy
* Corresponding author.
E-mail address: Gaetano.rocco@btopenworld.com

Thorac Surg Clin 20 (2010) 509–517
doi:10.1016/j.thorsurg.2010.09.001
1547-4127/10/$ — see front matter © 2010 Elsevier Inc. All rights reserved.

TIMING OF CHEST WALL INVOLVEMENT

Breast cancer may involve the chest wall during primary diagnosis (locally advanced breast cancer [LABC]) or later because of failure of BCT or a locoregional relapse after mastectomy.

LABC

The term LABC encompasses a wide array of breast tumors characterized by a high rate of locoregional relapses and heterogeneous differing prognostic outlook. Approximately 20% to 25% of overall breast cancers are locally advanced at the time of diagnosis.[10,11] According to the American Joint Committee on Cancer TNM staging system, all breast malignancies that are classified as T3 or T4 with any N subset or as N2 or N3 with any T subset are considered LABC.[12] Thus, all patients with stage III disease and some patients with stage IIB (T3-N0) meet the criteria for this classification.[13] **Table 1** summarizes the LABC classification. Patients with LABC often show a large breast mass associated with a wide locoregional lymphatic disease (large operable disease, **Fig. 1**). In some instances, the breast is diffusely involved and the chest wall is partially infiltrated (locally advanced disease, **Fig. 2**). Moreover, inflammatory breast cancer has a particularly aggressive pattern that falls under the heading of LABC, accounting for 1% to 3% of overall breast cancers.[14] Patients with inflammatory disease often present with erythema and edema of the skin (peau d'orange, **Fig. 3**) without an obvious mass within the breast.

Locoregional Breast Cancer Relapse

Locoregional breast cancer relapses (LRRs) are a heterogeneous group of lesions ranging from a small, solitary tumor nodule in the surgical scar to diffuse carcinoma *en cuirass* involving the entire chest wall and regional lymphatics. The incidence of LRR varies from 7% to 32% and depends on the initial extent of disease, the type of primary therapy, the length of follow-up, and the method of detection.[15] The condition in patients with advanced disease at the initial diagnosis recurs locally more rapidly than that in patients with early breast cancer at the initial diagnosis. From 60% to 80% of chest wall recurrences appear within the first 2 years after mastectomy, but local recurrence can occur throughout the patient's lifetime.[16]

Table 1
LABC classification according to the American Joint Committee on Cancer TMN staging system

LABC

T4 breast cancer: tumor of any size with direct extension to chest wall or skin

   T4a: extension to bone chest wall, including sternum, ribs, and clavicle

   T4b: edema (including peau d'orange) or ulceration of the skin of the breast or satellite skin nodules confined to the same breast

Locally advanced inflammatory breast carcinoma

N2b disease: metastasis only in ipsilateral internal mammary nodes and in the absence of axillary lymph node metastasis

N3 disease

   N3a: metastasis in ipsilateral infraclavicular lymph nodes

   N3b: metastasis in ipsilateral internal mammary lymph nodes and axillary lymph nodes

   N3c: metastasis in ipsilateral supraclavicular lymph nodes

Stage	Primary Tumor (T)	Regional Lymph Nodes (N)	Distant Metastases (M)
IIB	T3	N0	M0
IIIA	T0	N2	M0
	T1	N2	M0
	T2	N2	M0
	T3	N1	M0
	T3	N2	M0
IIIB	T4	Any N	M0
	Any T	N3	M0

Data from Woodward WA, Strom EA, Tucker SL, et al. Changes in the 2003 American Joint Committee on Cancer staging for breast cancer dramatically affect stage-specific survival. J Clin Oncol 2003;21(17):3244–8.

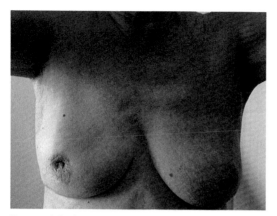

Fig. 1. Right large resectable breast carcinoma.

MECHANISMS OF CHEST WALL INVOLVEMENT BY BREAST CANCER

Breast cancer may involve the chest wall by direct infiltration or through regional lymphatic spreading. The tumor may infiltrate the following structures: skin, pectoral muscles, intercostal muscles, ribs, sternum, axillary and subclavian vessels, and the brachial plexus roots. Moreover, the cancer can spread across the ipsilateral regional lymphatics, such as axillary, infraclavicular, supraclavicular, and the internal mammary nodes. **Fig. 4** classifies the mechanisms of chest wall involvement by breast cancer depending on which structures are implicated.

Soft Tissue Chest Wall Involvement

Breast cancer may involve the skin of the anterior or anterolateral chest wall by direct infiltration (dermal infiltration, epidermis ulceration) or by

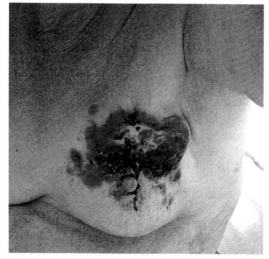

Fig. 2. Left locally advanced breast carcinoma.

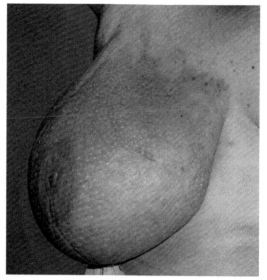

Fig. 3. Right inflammatory breast carcinoma.

subcutaneous lymphatic spreading (neoplastic lymphangitis, inflammatory carcinoma). Generally, the tumor may also infiltrate a partial segment of the pectoralis major muscle. In this case, resection of the portion involved after the line of the muscle fibers is indicated. Infrequently, the pectoral muscles may be extensively involved. In this case, both the pectoralis muscles must be sacrificed en bloc with the infraclavicular lymphatics.[17]

Axillary, Infraclavicular, and Supraclavicular Lymph Nodes Dissection

Breast cancer may involve the infraclavicular and supraclavicular lymph nodes in almost 5% of cases at primary diagnosis and in less than 2% of cases of regional recurrence.[18] The lymphadenectomy of the infraclavicular and the supraclavicular nodes should always be associated with the axillary dissection and with the resection of the interpectoral Rotter lymph nodes.[19] Exposure of the subclavian vessels and the infraclavicular lymph nodes can be widely obtained by dissecting the pectoralis minor muscle from the chest wall or, rarely, by removing the pectoralis minor muscle. Nevertheless, the exposure to the supraclavicular lymph nodes may not be sufficient, and hence, it is useful to divide the pectoralis major muscle at the level of the humeral insertion. This maneuver permits to overturn the muscle medially and to resect its clavicular attachment, thereby providing an access to the extrathoracic portion of the subclavian and axillary vessels as well as to the infra- and supraclavicular lymph nodes and the brachial plexus.[20]

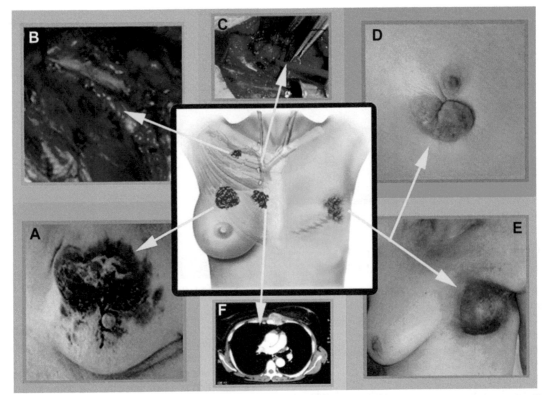

Fig. 4. Mechanisms of chest wall involvement by breast cancer (BC) depending on which structures are implicated. (*A*) BC involving the skin and the pectoralis major muscle. (*B*) BC infiltrating the subclavian vessels and/or involving the subclavian as well as the interpectoral Rotter lymph nodes. (*C*) BC involving the internal mammary chain. (*D*) BC locally recurred after mastectomy. (*E*) BC locally recurred after failure of BCT. (*F*) BC partially infiltrating the sternum and the ribs.

Resection of Axillary and Subclavian Vessels

Breast cancer can even involve the axillary and/or subclavian vessels. The mechanism implicated is almost always a bulky lymphatic metastasization. However, rare cases of direct tumor infiltration have been described. The exposure of the subclavian and axillary vessels is a critical point to perform a safe vascular dissection. The vessel wall can be resected tangentially and repaired with running suture. Moreover, the veins may be completely divided without reconstruction, whereas the arteries always require to be reconstructed. Revascularization is performed with an end-to-end anastomosis or, less frequently, by polytetrafluoroethylene graft (6–8 mm of diameter).[21] In these extraordinary rare cases, the transmanubrial surgical approach warrants sufficient exposure of the intrathoracic portion of the subclavian vessels, resulting in a safe vascular resection.[22]

Internal Mammary Lymph Node Dissection

The internal mammary lymph node involvement by breast cancer may be because of lymphatic spreading or may be associated with full-thickness chest wall infiltration. The lymphadenectomy of the internal mammary chain can be safely performed by video-assisted thoracoscopy or by using anterior mediastinoscopy or mediastinotomy.[23]

Full-Thickness Chest Wall Resection and Reconstruction

Breast cancer may infiltrate the intercostal muscles and the ribsas well as the sternum. In patients with this condition, the recommended surgical treatment is a full-thickness CWR. The excision should be performed on an area that includes approximately a 5-cm margin of healthy tissue around the tumor.[24] Shape, size, and site of the portion of chest wall involved are determinants in choosing the best surgical approach. The final goal is to radically resect the tumor en bloc with the infiltrated structures as well as to provide a reconstruction that results in a minimal paradox chest wall motion during respiration. Reconstruction is generally viewed as a procedure with 2 aspects, namely, chest wall stabilization and soft tissue reconstruction. However, in some cases, soft tissue reconstruction itself is sufficient to preserve the respiratory mechanics. The decision of whether chest wall stabilization is necessary relies on multiple factors, such as the size and composition of the defect, integrity and quality of the structures overlying the defect, and intrinsic qualities of the flaps used for soft tissue coverage. In addition, the patient's medical condition and ability to withstand a lengthy operative procedure as well as the patient's overall prognosis and desires must be considered.[25] Large defects almost always need some form of chest wall stabilization to preserve respiratory function. In particular, the anterior CWR owing to cancer involving multiple ribs and/or sternum requires stabilization with prosthetic material, even if the major pectorals muscle and the overlying skin and subcutaneous tissue are left intact. The materials used to stabilize the chest wall can be schematically classified into biologic and synthetic implants.[26] The advantages of autologous tissues are availability and biocompatibility. The drawbacks include poor resistance to infection, increased operating time, substantially increased patient discomfort, and relative flaccidity when compared with synthetic materials. Autologous bone grafts (tibia, fibula, and iliac crest) can be used judiciously in selected patients for chest wall reconstruction, although their harvesting adds another operative site with its associated comorbidities and potential complications.[26] Furthermore, preserved human or animal tissues have been mostly used with success for chest wall stabilization. However, the initial stability may become flaccid with time because of the peripheral stress on anchoring sutures as well as intrinsic weakening of structural proteins. Besides, the patient's body reacts to these materials as it does to any foreign body. Rarely, rejection occurs.[27] Most synthetic materials are available as sheets or as meshes (Marlex Mesh; Bard, Billerica, MA, USA; Prolene Mesh; Ethicon, Cinicinnati, OH, USA; Gore-Tex, Gore Dualmesh Plus Biomaterial; Gore, Flagstaff, AZ, USA). These materials can be used alone or in combination with methyl methacrylate monomer to increase the degree of firmness of the prosthesis.[28] Stabilization with either biologic or synthetic materials requires creative tailoring to customize the prosthesis and to stabilize the chest wall. In addition, the prosthesis requires to be covered by vital soft tissue. Usually, the soft tissue placed over the prosthesis is the residual native tissue at the site of the CWR, but in some cases a musculocutaneous flap is necessary for sufficient coverage. Pedicled reconstruction of chest wall defects may be performed on any anatomic region of the chest wall. Selection of appropriate flaps is mandatory because tension on a flap margin or its pedicle spells disaster. Coverage of the anterior or the anterolateral chest wall defects may be safely obtained using several pedicled flaps, such as pectoralis major, rectus abdominis, and latissimus dorsi as well as the omentum.[29] Occasionally, a defect may be so large that more than one flap may be necessary to provide for adequate soft tissue coverage. Each of the flaps used in reconstruction of the chest wall has advantages and drawbacks, and a high level of experience is necessary to individualize the reconstruction strategy.[30]

THE PREOPERATIVE WORKOUT

Candidates of CWR owing to breast cancer involvement require a full-staging workout, including history and physical examination, a complete blood cell count with biochemical survey (SMA-12) and tumor markers (cancer antigen 15.3 and carcinoembryonic antigen), chest radiography, mammography, breast and chest wall soft tissue ultrasonography, and magnetic resonance imaging (MRI) dynamic breast imaging. Bones scan and computed tomography of the chest, abdomen, and pelvis should rule out the presence of a distant metastatic disease.[31] Furthermore, the fludeoxyglucose F 18 positron emission tomography is useful to assess the locoregional lymph node involvement. Percutaneous core-biopsy or vacuum-assisted large gauge tumor biopsies with image guidance (ultrasonography and stereotactic or MRI guidance) are essential to confirm the diagnosis, leading to define important prognostic factors such as the histologic tumor type, grading, immunohistochemical hormone receptor status (estrogen receptor and progesterone receptor), and Her2/neu gene amplification and/or over expression.

THE SURGICAL PLAN

The management of the breast cancer involving chest wall remains a difficult clinical challenge because patients with this condition have high rates of local relapse and eventually die of metastatic disease. Therefore, these cases require a multidisciplinary approach and a multimodality treatment that includes induction chemotherapy, surgery, radiotherapy, and hormonal and targeted therapies.[32] The main goal of the surgical treatment is the best control of the locoregional disease, even if an extended CWR is necessary. Moreover, the CWR may be indicated to provide a good palliation and a better quality of life.[33]

The knowledge of locoregional extension of breast cancer through the chest wall is fundamental to choose the best surgical approach, assess which structures should be resected, and correctly plan the right reconstructive strategy. A case-by-case multidisciplinary approach is strongly recommended to elaborate the right surgical treatment. In fact, the heterogeneity of the clinical features makes it impossible to design one fixable surgical plan. The surgical team should be composed of the breast surgeon, thoracic surgeon, and plastic surgeon, whereas the orthopedic, vascular, and neurologic surgeons may be consulted on demand. The complex nature of these cases requires open communication between the ablative and the reconstructive teams to meet the oncologic target and preserve reconstructive options critical to successful closure of the defect.

REVIEW OF THE LITERATURE

The heterogeneity of clinical features showed by breast cancer involving the chest wall complicates the design of prospective randomized trials. Most studies have been small, single-centered and retrospective. Moreover, in these retrospective studies, patients present different stages at the time of diagnosis and receive different therapeutic approaches, making any comparison between studies difficult. The authors reviewed the literature specifically looking at the results of CWRs

for LABC as compared with those in which the resection was performed for recurrent breast cancer after mastectomy or after failure of BCT.

Results After CWR in LABC

Historically, patients with LABC have been treated with mastectomy if technically possible.[34] Failure of mastectomy alone to produce good survival rates prompted the use of systemic therapy. The hormonal therapy was introduced in the 1950s, whereas the chemotherapy was added in the 1970s.[35] In the 1980s, several studies demonstrated the ability of induction chemotherapy to convert some inoperable patients into candidates for mastectomy.[36] CWR was associated with mastectomy in almost 30% of patients. Perioperative mortality occurred in less then 2% of patients. Major and minor morbidities were observed in 10% and 30% of cases, respectively. **Table 2** summarizes the survival rates observed at 3 and 5 years in patients with stage III breast cancer treated with combined modality therapies.[37–46] The reported median survival rate for patients with LABC ranged from 28 to 66 months. Local recurrence was 7% in patients with stage IIIA cancer compared with 26% in those with stage IIIB disease. The 10-year disease-free survival (DFS) and OS rates for patients with stage IIIA breast cancer were 55% and 62%, respectively. However, the 10-year DFS and OS rates for

Table 2
Survival of stage III breast carcinoma after combined modality treatment

Authors	Year	Regimen	Number of Patients	3-Y Survival (%)	5-Y Survival (%)
De Lena et al[37]	1978	CT + RT ± S	110	50	NA
Bedwinek et al[38]	1982	CT + RT + CT	22	40	NA
Pawlicki et al[39]	1983	CT	40	13	NA
		CT + RT + CT	34	32	NA
		CT + S + RT + CT	13	62	NA
Valagussa et al[40]	1983	CT + RT	72	43	20
		CT + RT + CT	126	60	36
		CT + S + CT	79	64	49
Conte et al[41]	1987	CT + S + CT	39	60	NA
Hortobagyi et al[42]	1988	CT ± S + RT	174	65	55
Touboul et al[43]	1992	CT + RT + CT ± S + CT	82	85	81
Low et al[44]	2004	CT ± S + RT	107	NA	38[a]
Huang et al[45]	2008	CT ± S ± RT	542	NA	54[a]
Frasci et al[46]	2010	CT + S + RT	200	91 vs 78	82 vs 69

Abbreviations: CT, chemotherapy; NA, not available; RT, radiotherapy; S, surgery.
[a] Ten-year survival.

Table 3
Literature review of OS after curative CWR for locoregional breast cancer recurrence

Study	Number of Patients	5-Y Survival (%)	Local Control (%)	Prognostic Factors
Kluiber et al[49]	12	27	NA	NA
Soysal et al[50]	10	33	NA	NA
Faneyte et al[51]	30	45	NA	Age 35 y, interval 2 y
Toi et al[52]	15	47	NA	Interval 5 y
Ohuchi et al[53]	16	57	NA	Interval 5 y
Kolodziejski et al[54]	13	62	NA	NA
Miyauchi et al[55]	23	48	56 (5 y)	NA
Pfannschmidt et al[56]	33	41	85 (3y)	Interval 2 y, no adjuvant chemotherapy
Downey et al[57]	38	18	NA	Initial node status
Warzelhan et al[58]	22	71	NA	NA
Pameijer et al[59]	22	71	NA	NA
van der Pol et al[60]	77	25	82 (5 y)	Interval, chemotherapy before CWR, tumor size

[a] Univariate analysis.
[b] Multivariate interval 10 years.
   Data from van der Pol CC, van Geel AN, Menke-Pluymers MB, et al. Prognostic factors in 77 curative chest wall resections for isolated breast cancer recurrence. Ann Surg Oncol 2009;16(12):3414–21.

patients with stage IIIB disease were 30% and 31%, respectively. Lymphatic involvement was probably the most important prognostic factor, and the survival rates depended, in part, on the number of involved nodes. Valagussa and colleagues[40] showed a 5-years survival rate of 49% for patients with N0 disease, 40% for those with N1 disease, and 17% for those with N2 disease. Moreover, the size of the tumor had a prognostic significance. These investigators reported 5-year survival rates of 65% for patients with tumors less than 5 cm in diameter, 36% for those with tumors 5 to 10 cm, and 16% for those with tumors larger than 10 cm. Also, the estrogen receptor positivity was associated with a significantly longer DFS time and higher OS rate, especially among patients with operable disease.[36] Other prognostic factors that correlated with a better prognosis were the operability of the tumor at the time of primary diagnosis, grade of response to the induction chemotherapy, and completeness of surgical resection.[46]

Results After CWR for Locoregional Breast Cancer Recurrence

In 1907, Sauerbruch[47] reported the first extensive CWR for locally recurrent breast carcinoma. Maier[48] revived the procedure in 1947. Later, several larger series have shown that CWR is a safe and justifiable procedure with relatively low mortality

(0% to 5%) and morbidity.[49–60] The integration of chemotherapy, surgery, and radiotherapy in a multimodality treatment plan has drastically improved the control of the local disease as well as the OS. The reported 5-year OS rate ranges from 40% to 60% from the time of recurrence, and the DFS at 5 years varies from 26% to 67%. **Table 3** summarizes the larger series reported in the literature.[49–60] The type of local recurrence portends no prognostic difference. Only a few of the larger series report the rate of pathologically confirmed radical resection after CWR. In these series, the correlation between R1 and R0 resection and DFS or OS was not significant. This was probably the result of postoperative radiotherapy in patients with an R1 resection. On the other hand, the age of the patient at the time of the diagnosis and the interval between initial treatment and CWR of 2 years or 5 years were described as statistically significant negative prognostic factors for OS and DFS.

SUMMARY

Chest wall involvement by breast cancer remains a difficult clinical challenge that may occur at the time of the primary diagnosis (LABC) or later as a result of locoregional breast cancer recurrence. A case-by-case multidisciplinary approach is strongly recommended, and a multimodality therapy should be always considered. Full-thickness resection of the chest wall can be done with acceptable morbidity and mortality, providing a good palliation and a better quality of life even to patients with poor prognosis. Moreover, in well-selected cases, CWR results in locoregional control of disease and prolongation of life.

REFERENCES

1. Ferlay J, Bray F, Pisani P, et al. Globocan 2002. Cancer incidence, mortality and prevalence worldwide. IARC CancerBase No. 5, version 2.0. Lyon (France): IARCPress; 2004.

2. American Cancer Society breast cancer facts & figures, 2005–2006.

3. Young JL Jr, Roffers SD, Ries LA, et al, editors. SEER summary staging manual—2001: codes and coding instructions. Bethesda (MD): National Cancer Institute; 2001. p. 185–205. NIH Pub. No.01–4969.

4. Horner MJ, Ries LAG, Krapcho M, et al, editors. SEER cancer statistics review, 1975–2006. Bethesda (MD): National Cancer Institute; 2006.

5. Fisher B, Anderson S, Bryant J, et al. Twenty-year follow-up of a randomized trial comparing total mastectomy, lumpectomy, and lumpectomy plus irradiation for the treatment of invasive breast cancer. N Engl J Med 2002;347(16):1233–41.

6. Blichert-Toft M, Rose C, Andersen JA, et al. Danish randomized trial comparing breast conservation therapy with mastectomy: six years of life-table analysis. Danish breast cancer cooperative group. J Natl Cancer Inst Monogr 1992;11:19–25.

7. Van Dongen JA, Bartelink H, Fentiman IS, et al. Randomized clinical trial to assess the value of breast-conserving therapy in stage I and II breast cancer, EORTC 10801 trial. J Natl Cancer Inst Monogr 1992;11:15–8.

8. Jacobson JA, Danforth DN, Cowan KH, et al. Ten-year results of a comparison of conservation with mastectomy in the treatment of stage I and II breast cancer. N Engl J Med 1995;332(14):907–11.

9. Veronesi U, Cascinelli N, Mariani L, et al. Twenty-year follow-up of a randomized study comparing breast-conserving surgery with radical mastectomy for early breast cancer. N Engl J Med 2002; 347(16):1227–32.

10. Singletary SE, Allred C, Ashley P, et al. Revision of the American Joint Committee on cancer staging system for breast cancer. J Clin Oncol 2002; 20(17):3628–36.

11. Woodward WA, Strom EA, Tucker SL, et al. Changes in the 2003 American Joint Committee on cancer staging for breast cancer dramatically affect stage-specific survival. J Clin Oncol 2003;21(17):3244–8.

12. Harris J. Staging of breast cancer. In: Harris J, editor. Disease of the breast. 2nd edition. Philadelphia: Lippincott Williams & Wilkins; 2000. p. 562–5.

13. Jaiyesimi IA, Budzar AU, Hortobagyi G. Inflammatory breast cancer: a review. J Clin Oncol 1992;10: 1014.

14. Martin JK, van Heerden JA, Gattey TA. Synchronous and metachronous carcinoma of the breast. Surgery 1982;91:12.

15. Medino-Franco H, van Heerden JA, Gaffey TA. Factors associated with local recurrence after skin-sparing mastectomy and immediate breast reconstruction for invasive breast cancer. Ann Surg 2002;235:814.

16. Stelzer D, Gay WA. Tumors of the chest wall. Surg Clin North Am 1980;60:779.

17. Clemons M, Danson S, Hamilton T, et al. Locoregional recurrent breast cancer: incidence, risk factors and survival. Cancer Treat Rev 2001;27:67.

18. Wickerham DL, Fisher B. Surgical treatment of primary breast cancer. Semin Surg Oncol 1988;4: 226.

19. Hathaway CL, Rand MP, Moe R, et al. Salvage surgery for locally advanced and locally recurrent breast cancer. Arch Surg 1994;129:582.

20. Freedman GM, Anderson PR, Li T, et al. Locoregional recurrence of triple-negative breast cancer after breast-conserving surgery and radiation. Cancer 2009;115(5):946–51.

21. Fadel E, Chapelier A, Carrina J, et al. Subclavian artery and reconstruction for thoracic inlet cancers. J Vasc Surg 1999;28:581.

22. Veronesi G, Scanagatta P, Goldhirsch A, et al. Results of chest wall resection for recurrent or locally advanced breast malignancies. Breast 2007;16(3): 297–302.

23. Ogawa Y, Ishikawa T, Ikeda K, et al. The thoracoscopic approach for internal mammary nodes 186 in breast cancer. Surg Endosc 2000;14:1149–52.

24. El-Tamer M, Chaglassian T, Martini N. Resection and debridement of chest wall tumors and general aspects of reconstruction. Surg Clin North Am 1989;69:947.

25. Seyfer AE, Graeber GM, Wind GG. Planning the reconstruction. In: Seyer AE, editor. Atlas of chest wall reconstruction. Rockville (MD): Aspen Publishers; 1986. p. 134–6.

26. Boyd AD, Shaw WW, McCarthy JC, et al. Immediate reconstruction of full-thickness chest wall defects. Ann Thorac Surg 1993;91:828.

27. McCormark PM, Bains MS, Beattie EJ, et al. New trends in skeletal reconstruction after resection of chest wall tumors. Ann Thorac Surg 1981;31:45.

28. McCormark PM. Use of prosthetic materials in chest wall reconstruction: assets and liabilities. Surg Clin North Am 1989;69:965.

29. Seyfer AE, Graeber GM, Wind GG. The pectoralis major muscle and the musculocutaneous flaps. In: Seyer AE, editor. Atlas of chest wall reconstruction. Rockville (MD): Aspen Publishers; 1986. p. 186–91.

30. Rocco G, Fazioli F, La Manna C, et al. Omental flap and titanium plates provide structural stability and protection of the mediastinum after extensive sternocostal resection. Ann Thorac Surg 2010;90: e14–6.

31. Azarow KS, Mallow M, Seyer AE, et al. Preoperative evaluation and general preparation for chest wall operations. Surg Clin North Am 1989;69:899.

32. Hunt KK, Ames FC, Singletary SE. Locally advanced noninflammatory breast cancer. Surg Clin North Am 1996;76:393.

33. Brito RA, Valero V, Buzdar AU, et al. Long-term results of combined-modality therapy for locally advanced breast cancer with ipsilateral supraclavicular metastases: the University of Texas M.D. Anderson Cancer Center experience. J Clin Oncol 2001; 19:628.

34. Haagensen C, Stout A. Carcinoma of the breast II: criteria of inoperability. Ann Surg 1943;118:1032.

35. Derman DP, Browde S, Kessel IL, et al. Adjuvant chemotherapy (CMF) for stage III breast cancer: a randomized trial. Int J Radiat Oncol Biol Phys 1989;17:257.

36. Perloff M, Lesnick GJ. Chemotherapy before and after mastectomy in stage III breast cancer. Arch Surg 1982;117:879.

37. De Lena M, Zucali R, Vigliotti G. Combined chemotherapy radiotherapy approach in locally advanced breast cancer. Cancer Chemother Pharmacol 1978; 1:53.

38. Bedwinek J, Rao DV, Perez C, et al. Stage III and localized stage IV breast cancer: irradiation alone versus irradiation plus surgery. Int J Radiat Oncol Biol Phys 1982;8:31.

39. Pawlicki M, Skolyszewski J, Brandys A. Results of combined treatment of patients with locally advanced breast cancer (IIIA-IIIB). Tumori 1983;69:249.

40. Valagussa P, Zambetti M, Bignami P, et al. T3b-T4 breast cancer: factors affecting results in combined modality treatments. Clin Exp Metastasis 1983;1:191.

41. Conte PF, Alama A, Bartelli G, et al. Chemotherapy with estrogenic recruitment and surgery in locally advanced breast cancer: clinical and cytokinetic results. Int J Cancer 1987;40:490.

42. Hortobagyi GN, Amez FC, Buzdar AU, et al. Management of stage III primary breast cancer with primary chemotherapy, surgery, and radiotherapy. Cancer 1988;62:2507.

43. Touboul E, Lefranc JP, Blondon J, et al. Multidisciplinary treatment approach to locally advanced noninflammatory breast cancer using chemotherapy and radiotherapy with or without surgery. Radiother Oncol 1992;25:167.

44. Low JA, Berman AW, Steinberg SM, et al. Long-term follow-up for locally advanced and inflammatory breast cancer patients treated with multimodality therapy. J Clin Oncol 2004;22(20):4067–74.

45. Huang EH, Liao Z, Cox JD, et al. Comparison of outcomes for patients with unresectable, locally advanced non-small-cell lung cancer treated with induction chemotherapy followed by concurrent chemoradiation vs. concurrent chemoradiation alone. Int J Radiat Oncol Biol Phys 2007;68(3):779–85.

46. Frasci G, D'Aiuto G, Comella P, et al. Preoperative weekly cisplatin, epirubicin, and paclitaxel (PET) improves prognosis in locally advanced breast cancer patients: an update of the Southern Italy cooperative oncology group (SICOG) randomised trial 99. Ann Oncol 2010;21(4):707–16.

47. Sauerbruch F. Beitrag zur resection der brustwant mit plastick auf die freigelecte lunge. Deutsch Z Chir 1907;86:275–80 [in German].

48. Maier HC. Surgical management of large defects of the thoracic wall. Surgery 1947;22(2):169–78.

49. Kluiber R, Bines S, Bradley C, et al. Major chest wall resection for recurrent breast carcinoma. Am Surg 1991;57:523–9.

50. Soysal O, Wallsh CI, Nesbitt JC, et al. Resection of sternal tumors: extent, reconstruction, and survival. Ann Thorac Surg 1995;60:1353–8.

51. Faneyte IF, Rutgers EJ, Zoetmulder FA. Chest wall resection in the treatment of locally recurrent breast carcinoma: indications and outcome for 44 patients. Cancer 1997;80:886–91.

52. Toi M, Tanaka S, Bando M, et al. Outcome of surgical resection for chest wall recurrence in breast cancer patients. J Surg Oncol 1997;64:23–6.

53. Ohuchi N, Hirakawa H, Abe M. Full thickness chest wall resection for recurrent breast cancer with reference to prognostic factors. Nippon Geka Gakkai Zasshi 1993;94:745–50.

54. Kolodziejski LS, Wysocky WM, Komorowski AL. Full-thickness chest wall resection for recurrence of breast malignancy. Breast J 2005;11:273–7.

55. Miyauchi K, Koyama H, Noguchi S, et al. Surgical treatment for chest wall recurrence of breast cancer. Eur J Cancer 1992;28A:1059–62.

56. Pfannschmidt J, Geisbusch P, Muley T, et al. Surgical resection of secondary chest wall tumors. Thorac Cardiovasc Surg 2005;53:234–9.

57. Downey RJ, Rush V, Hsu FI, et al. Chest wall resection for locally recurrent breast cancer: is it worthwhile? J Thorac Cardiovasc Surg 2000;119:420–8.

58. Warzelhan J, Stoelben E, Imdahl A, et al. Results in surgery for primary and metastatic chest wall tumors. Eur J Cardiothorac Surg 2001;19:584–8.

59. Pameijer CR, Smith D, McCahill LE, et al. Full-thickness chest wall resection for recurrent breast carcinoma: an institutional review and meta-analysis. Am Surg 2005;71:711–5.

60. van der Pol CC, van Geel AN, Menke-Pluymers MB, et al. Prognostic factors in 77 curative chest wall resections for isolated breast cancer recurrence. Ann Surg Oncol 2009;16:3414–21.

Non–Small Cell Lung Cancer Invading the Chest Wall

Marc Riquet, MD, PhD*, Alex Arame, MD,
Françoise Le Pimpec Barthes, MD, PhD

KEYWORDS

- Non–small cell lung cancer • Chest wall reconstruction
- T3 • N2 • Neoadjuvant therapy • Adjuvant therapy

Once a surgical challenge with a dismal prognosis, non–small cell lung cancer (NSCLC) invading the chest wall (CW) was considered not amenable to surgery. However, the feasibility of surgery providing good results was demonstrated in 1947.[1] Nowadays, resecting part of the CW, whatever its extent or location, is no longer a technical problem, as demonstrated elsewhere in this review.

INCIDENCE OF CW INVASION

The CW is invaded by lung cancer in about 5% of the resected patients,[2] and is thus obviously more frequent than primary CW tumors invading the lung. It represented 125 out of 1590 (7.9%) patients who underwent pulmonary resection for NSCLC,[3] and 125 out of the 275 patients (45.5%) classified as pT3 in the former TNM classification of Mountain.[4] The other pT3 includes tumors of the main bronchus less than 2 cm from the carina and tumors invading the diaphragm, the mediastinal pleura, and the pericardium.

In the new TNM classification,[5] NSCLC invading the CW is still classified as T3, with no staging modification. However, the pT3 group now also includes tumors measuring more than 7 cm and tumors with presence of an other nodule in the same lobe. Accordingly, the incidence of CW invasion might change in the pT3 subgroup in the next available data. In the authors' practice (Marc Riquet, MD, PhD, unpublished data, 2009), pT3 represents 1074 of 4471 patients with resected NSCLC (24%). Among pT3 tumors, tumors with CW invasion represent 32.2% (346/1074), tumors larger than 7 cm 20.9% (225/1074), and tumors with nodule in the same lobe 10.4% (112/1074).

In any event, the prognosis of the tumors with CW invasion is the same as the prognosis of any other resected NSCLC regardless of its pT, mainly depending on the completeness of resection and on the presence of lymph node (LN) involvement, and more particularly on the degree of this LN involvement.

GROSS PATHOLOGY CHARACTERISTICS

The CW invasion generally originates from peripheral tumors and takes place progressively. The tumor first invades the parietal pleura and progresses deeper as the time passes, to soft tissue and intercostal muscles, and finally the ribs. Frequency of tissue involvement in depth progression is shown in **Table 1**.[3,6–14]

When the tumor infiltrates the soft tissue, muscles, or bones, a complete CW resection, that is, encompassing intercostal spaces, ribs, and sometimes extrathoracic muscles, is necessary to achieve a radical operation. When the tumor has only penetrated the parietal pleura, an extrapleural resection avoiding resection of ribs and muscles may be considered. In effect, the sub(parietal) pleural endothoracic fascia makes up a natural barrier to the cancer invasion, and the parietal pleura and endothoracic fascia are usually involved by an "adhering" more than an "infiltrating" process. Consequently, some of

Department of Thoracic Surgery, Georges Pompidou European Hospital, 20 rue Leblanc, 75015, Paris, France
* Corresponding author.
E-mail address: marc.riquet@egp.aphp.fr

Thorac Surg Clin 20 (2010) 519–527
doi:10.1016/j.thorsurg.2010.06.004

Table 1
Chest wall invasion according to parietal pleura, soft tissue and muscle, ribs, and 5-year survival rates

Study	Year	No. of Patients	Pleura	Muscle	Ribs	5-yr Extra Pleura	5-yr Pleura Chest Wall	5-yr Muscle	5-yr Ribs
Chapelier et al[6]	2000	100	29 (29%)	67 (67%)	24 (24%)	None	na[a]	na	na
Facciolo et al[7]	2001	104	28 (26.9%)	36 (36.6%)	40 (38.5%)	None	79%	52.1%	53.4%
Magdeleinat et al[8]	2001	201	89 (44.3%)	112 (55.7%)		37%	31%	15%	na
Elia et al[9]	2001	110	63 (69.3%)	47 (30.7%)		na	na	na	na
Burkhart et al[10]	2002	95	29 (30.5%)	43 (45.3%)	23 (24.2%)	0	49.9%	35%	31.6%
Riquet et al[3]	2002	125	44 (35.2%)	45 (36%)	36 (28.8%)	14.4%		25.7%	26.1%
Akay et al[11]	2002	85	29 (34.1%)	56 (65.9%)		None	33%	17%	na
Matsuoka et al[12]	2004	76	40 (52.6%)	10 (13.2%)	26 (34.2%)	30%	32.5%	30%	38.5%
Doddoli et al[13]	2005	309	158 (51.1%)	75 (24.3%)	76 (24.6%)	39.1%	60.3%	41%	31.8%
Lin et al[14]	2006	42	11 (26.2%)	31 (73.8%)		None	10.9%	33.5%	na

Abbreviations: na, not available; None, no extrapleural resection was performed.

[a] Extension to the parietal pleura only, was associated with a significant increase in long-term survival when compared with deeper involvement (*P* value 0.02 and 0.024 in uni- and multivariate analysis, respectively).

these tumors may be detached from the bony CW by extrapleural dissection.[9]

The size of the tumor, its contact surface with the CW, and the pathologic depth of its invasion may vary from one patient to another, and are not necessary related. A large tumor may have a small depth of invasion despite needing a large CW resection. By contrast, a small tumor may be cured by a limited CW resection while deeply invading the CW. The authors were unable to find in the literature whether this discrepancy between tumor size and depth of CW invasion has a relevant prognostic value.

Besides the size and the depth of invasion, the tumor location has technical importance. The location may be posterior, lateral, or anteromedial. Posteriorly located tumors may be observed in 36.2% to 46% of patients,[9,15] of which many arise from the apicoposterior part of the upper or lower lobe of the lungs. The CW resection does not present any difficulty in the case of the lung cancers invading CW anteriorly to the midaxillary line. By contrast, some posteriorly located tumors tend to infiltrate the paravertebral portions of the ribs. Such invasion may compromise the possibility of resection in the case of tumors invading the vertebral bodies (thereby becoming pT4). The most frequent tumor of this type is the Pancoast tumor. A Pancoast tumor is located in the apex of the thorax and is classified as T4 in the new TNM classification, if there is evidence of invasion of the vertebral body or spinal canal, encasement of the subclavian vessels, or unequivocal involvement of the superior branches of the brachial plexus (C8 or above). In the absence of these conditions, the tumor is classified as T3.[5] Pancoast tumor surgery is generally dealt with in separate book chapters when T4, but these tumors share the same characteristics as others invading the CW when remaining purely T3.

COMPLETENESS OF RESECTION

The completeness of the tumor resection depends on the characteristics of the CW involvement. Macroscopic (R2) incomplete resection may be observed in the case of extension toward the vertebral column, and microscopic (R1) ones in the case of extension toward the paravertebral sulcus. R1 disease may be difficult to assess by the pathologist in case of CW resection because of the difficulties in analyzing all margins. Immunohistochemical analysis may help to identify microscopic tumor spread of the resection margins and patients at higher risk of recurrence,[16] but this is not the common practice. Microscopic R1 resection may also be the consequence of extrapleural

resection performed for tumors that seem to be only invading the parietal pleura, but actually infiltrate beyond the endothoracic fascia. Both R2 and R1 resections are not infrequent, ranging from 17.4% (34/195)[8] to 21.6% (21/97),[12] significantly decreasing the 5-year survival rates to 13% and 14.3%, respectively.

Thus, R2 and R1 CW resection dramatically worsens the prognosis, and should be avoided. Many studies do not include them in their report,[3,7,10,13,14,17] or only report the R0 and R1 resections.[6,11] This raises the question of how to detect whether the parietal pleura and the CW are infiltrated, not only to assess the diagnosis but also to foresee resection incompleteness, in order to prevent its risk by resorting multimodality treatments or definitely precluding surgery.

CW INVASION PREOPERATIVE DIAGNOSIS

Tumors with potential CW involvement do not generally require any specialized imaging, and the patients can proceed directly to surgery after careful nodal and systemic staging.[18] Visible rib destruction or infiltration of the soft tissue is a very specific sign for CW invasion (**Fig. 1**), any discovering CW invasion does not contraindicate CW resection. Inversely, the tumors in contact with the CW do not always directly invade the adjacent structures and are commonly T1 or T2 tumors. Thoracic surgeons are familiar with the low correlation between radiologic and pathologic findings in this subject area.[18] The T compartment is more often clinically overstaged than understaged. The important point is to anticipate the true depth of invasion in order to avoid incomplete extrapleural resection in the case of parietal pleura invasion and incomplete full CW resection in the case of paravertebral sulcus invasion.

In the case of paravertebral sulcus tumor, incomplete resection may occur by failing to recognize vertebral (T4) or paravertebral foramen invasion. When tumors are potentially invading the thoracic vertebrae, magnetic resonance imaging (MRI) may prove helpful by demonstrating intraforaminal invasion or by disclosing epiduritis.[19] Simultaneous presence of epiduritis and vertebral invasion may be considered as a contraindication to surgery, whereas vertebral foramen or body invasion can be addressed by a combined surgical approach in selected patients.

In the case of parietal pleural invasion, preoperative assessment leading directly to CW resection is difficult and may be nonconclusive. The combination of 2 or 3 criteria such as a tumor with more than 3 cm of surface contact with the pleura,

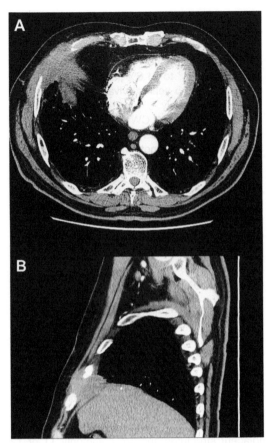

Fig. 1. Computed tomodensitometry demonstrating chest wall invasion including soft tissue and ribs (*A*) and lateral view (*B*).

obtuse angle, and associated pleural thickening comprises good, sensitive, but not specific information toward determining CW invasion. Obliteration of the extrapleural fat pad is a more sensitive and specific finding than thickening of the pleura.[20,21] However, limitations and low accuracy of static computed tomography (CT) scan or MRI have been highlighted,[22] and even high-resolution CT scan, or ultrasonography (US) may not help answer the question of whether the parietal pleura and CW are infiltrated or not.[17,22,23] Respiratory dynamic (RD) MRI may add much. Demonstrating the independent movement of the CW and lungs during breathing may help rule out parietal pleural invasion; RD-MRI has a sensitivity of 100% and specificity of 82.9% as a result of possible presence of inflammatory dense adhesions. Similar evaluation of the CW invasion has been reported using US.[22,24] Sensitivity and specificity were reported to be 100% and 98%, respectively. However, tumors near the vertebrae or apex were considered difficult to assess because of the

acoustic shadow of the bones and limited tumor movement during breathing. US-examination accuracy is also a highly operator-dependent procedure. RD-US proved to be more sensitive than CT scanning,[23] but in any case, RD-US only discriminates between parietal pleura tumor adhesion and contact without adhesion, but does not indicate whether the adhesion is tumoral or inflammatory. Thus, the decision of performing extrapleural or en bloc CW resection is still most often made intraoperatively by the surgeon.

CW RESECTION

A posterolateral thoracic approach for resecting NSCLC invading the CW is sufficient in most cases; however, for cancers invading the CW anteriorly near the sternum, an anterolateral or anterior approach may be advisable.[2] In any event it is important to open the chest far enough from the involved area, and then carefully palpate the CW and the tumor to determine whether there is true adhesion and to circumscribe the contours.[25] The security margin that was respected in some series is not always mentioned.[3,8–10,12] Some investigators recommend resecting one segment of the intact rib above and below the gross margin of the tumor and at least 3[6] to 4 cm[7] laterally. Akay and colleagues[11] report resecting a 4-cm margin of normal tissue on all sides, without recommending that their margin for tumors extend toward the vertebral column. In fact, the CW should be resected with at least 1.0 cm margin in all directions (**Fig. 2**).[25] A frozen section of the CW margins is not used routinely because of difficulty in evaluating such large specimens and bony structures, but may be useful on precisely indicated nonbony doubtful areas. In the case of NSCLC abutting the paravertebral sulcus, it may be necessary to disarticulate the ribs from the vertebrae. During this procedure, intercostal arteries may be injured at the level of the dorsal branches, whose spinal ramifications provide blood supply to the spinal cord.[26] The spinal cord vascularization may therefore be endangered. It is advisable to check the presence of spinal cord artery by means of medullary arteriography when suspected.

In the case of parietal pleural invasion, some investigators systematically remove the CW.[6,7,10] In some reports, no difference has been reported in the results of extrapleural resection and en bloc CW resection.[8,9,11,12] Akay and colleagues[11] found similar 5-year survival rates between patients who underwent extrapleural resection for limited parietal pleura invasion and CW resection for deeper CW invasion. Doddoli and colleagues[13] found a better prognosis when en

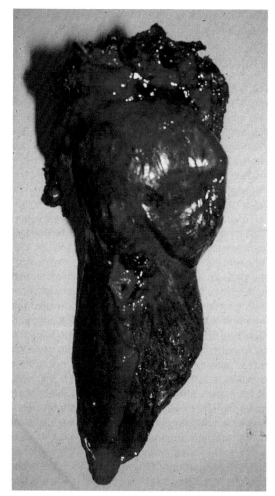

Fig. 2. An en bloc chest wall and lung resection (left upper lobe), and security margins.

bloc resection was performed. Thus, whether surgeons should perform an extra pleural resection or an en bloc CW resection when the tumor invades the pleura still remains a matter of debate. Moreover, microscopic invasion may extend beyond elastic fibers of the visceral pleura without penetration to the parietal pleura at tight adhesion sites, and discriminating between such T2-T3 forms may be impossible for the surgeon. The prognosis of this subgroup is reported to be identical to the prognosis of T2 NSCLC,[27] and does not justify en bloc CW resection.

REPLACEMENT OF THE CW

Small posterior defects less than 3.0 cm in diameter or those that are covered by the scapula do not usually necessitate CW reconstruction. Reconstruction is performed for defects of 3 or more ribs, unless covered by the scapula,

therefore defects outside of the area of coverage of the scapula often need to be reconstructed. However, when the defect is located at the tip of the scapula, a reconstruction is recommended to avoid entrapment of the scapula on the edge of the CW resection.[25] In such cases, the authors also currently perform a scapular tip resection, which aids in preventing the scapular entrapment. The need for reconstruction is variable and is reported as representing 40%,[13] 50%,[8] and 64%[10,11] of CW resections.

The use of rigid prosthesis is not recommended because rigid materials tend, due to continuous respiratory movements, to break and penetrate the surrounding tissue.[2] The most frequent alternative for CW reconstruction is polypropylene mesh, polyglactin 910 mesh (**Fig. 3**), or polytetrafluoroethylene. Autologous muscle flap transposition also covers the CW defect. The method is systematically used by Facciolo and colleagues,[7] and reported to be used in 25 out of 61 reconstructions by Magdeleinat and colleagues[8] (either isolated or in association) and 20 out of 36 reconstructions by Akay and colleagues.[11] In reality, most investigators resort to the flexible prosthesis (**Fig. 4**).

COMPLICATIONS

The mean of postoperative mortality is about 6%, ranging from 0% to 7.8%.[7–10,13] In hospital, death was reported by Martin-Ucar and colleagues[15] to complicate 7.3% of CW resections, but was still more important when 60-day mortality was considered (up to 19%). Mortality is mainly caused by respiratory problems or failure with frequency, ranging from 66% to 75%,[2,13,15] and may be estimated to be 3 times more frequent than for resections without CW.[2] The possibility of paradoxical movements of the chest wall after extensive resections may aggravate postoperative physiologic

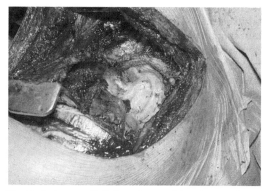

Fig. 3. A chest wall defect after en bloc chest wall and lung resection (left upper lobe).

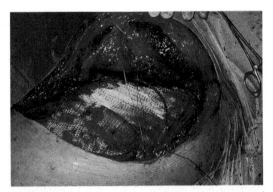

Fig. 4. A chest wall defect replacement by means of flexible prosthesis.

consequences.[28] The factors rendering patients highly susceptible to pulmonary complications leading to increased mortality are advanced age, limited respiratory reserve, and significant weight loss. The reversible factors must be addressed before performing en bloc pulmonary and CW resection for NSCLC. Another serious complication related to surgery is local infection that may lead to the ablation of the prosthetic material, which is the most important way for controlling the infection with a foreign body in place.[25] If sufficient time has elapsed since the resection, a fibrous scar would be formed, preventing the underlying lung from collapsing or paradoxic motion. The other serious complication, which must always be kept in mind, is paraplegia following costovertebral disarticulation in the case of tumors invading the paravertebral sulcus.[26] Its probability is rare but requires patient acknowledgement.

RESULTS

Long-term results are good (see **Table 1**). Local recurrences represent 12.5% to 30% of all recurrences,[3,6,11,12] many of them being associated with distant metastases. Local recurrence may be as low as 1.1% (1 out of 96 patients).[7] When the resection is complete, the number of resected ribs does not generally seem to be a prognostic factor,[7,9,11,12] or does not play any role. However, several resected ribs superior to 2 were sometimes found to be an indicator of poor prognosis.[6,13] CW resection permits good local control, and also plays an important, although most often forgotten role in quality of life by reducing pain. Indeed, pain is the principal clinical sign that leads patients to consult,[9] as a highly specific (>90%) clinical sign for CW infiltration.[2] Elia and colleagues[9] reported that the resolution of pain was achieved in all patients after CW

resection, and stressed its palliative as well as curative effect.

N2 INVOLVEMENT

N2 involvement generally indicates a poor prognosis. N2 frequency and survival rates vary from one series to another (**Table 2**). The frequency of N2 involvement is not related to the depth of CW invasion, even if a tendency to small differences seems to exist between parietal pleura and deeper invasion (**Table 3**). In the series of Akay and colleagues,[11] who found similar 5-year survival rates between patients who underwent extrapleural resection for limited parietal pleura invasion and CW resection for deeper invasion, pN positive involvement was observed in 31% and 21.4%, respectively. In the study by Lin and colleagues,[14] the patients with soft tissue or bone invasion had a tendency toward better 5-year survival rates than patients with only parietal pleura invasion. It was noted that patients with parietal pleura invasion had more N positive involvement than the other patients. Others also reported lesser survival rates,[3] and the patients also showed important N positive involvement rates. However, in both studies the differences were not significant. If such differences exist, they should probably occur because patients with major T3N2 are certainly rarely referred for surgical intervention.

For many investigators, the histologic proof of N2 involvement should lead to the recommendation of nonsurgical treatment such as radiotherapy and chemotherapy,[2] or at least to chemotherapy or radiotherapy + chemotherapy, either as induction or definitive treatment.[25] N2 disease is effectively a strong indicator for distant metastatic disease.[18] However, Magdeleinat and colleagues[8] reported that before 1990, they judged patients with suspicion of limited N2 disease as immediately operable, and that thereafter the patients with enlarged mediastinal N2 underwent mediastinoscopy. If N2 was confirmed, neoadjuvant chemotherapy was administered. Patients underwent surgery if objective response or no progression was observed, provided that the whole disease was judged resectable. These investigators reported encouraging results (see **Table 2**), which are paving the way for resorting to neoadjuvant therapy rather than systematically precluding surgery.

PREOPERATIVE HISTOPATHOLOGIC DIAGNOSIS

Preoperative diagnosis is essential for planning the appropriate treatment policy. Because other

Table 2
Chest wall invasion and N involvement

Study	Year	No. of Patients	N0	N1	N2	5-yr N0	5-yr N1	5-yr N2	5-yr Overall
Chapelier et al[6]	2000	100	65 (65%)	28 (28%)	7 (7%)	22%	9%	0%	18%
Facciolo et al[7]	2001	104	83 (79.8%)	5 (4.8%)	16 (15.4%)	67.3%	100%	17.9%	61.4%
Magdeleinat et al[8]	2001	195[a]	116 (58%)	52 (26%)	27 (13%)	25%	20%	21%	21%
Elia et al[9]	2001	110	83 (75.5%)	17 (15.5%)	10 (9%)	40%	0%	0%	?
Burkhart et al[10]	2002	95	65 (68.4%)	16 (16.8%)	14 (14.8%)	44.3%	26.3%	38.7%	38.7%
Riquet et al[3]	2002	125	77 (61.6%)	13 (10.4%)	35 (28%)	30.5%	0%	11.5%	22.5%
Akay et al[11]	2002	85	64 (75.3%)	12 (14.1%)	9 (10.6%)	na	na	na	na
Matsuoka et al[12]	2004	76	43 (52.6%)	15 (13.2%)	19[b] (34.2%)	44.2%	40%	6.2%	34.2%
Doddoli et al[13]	2005	309	212 (68.6%)	32 (10.4%)	65 (21%)	40%	23.8%	8.4%	30.7%
Lin et al[14]	2006	42	28 (67.6%)	14 (32.4%)	65 (21%)	39%	17.1%	28.4%	28.4%

Abbreviation: na, not available.
[a] Six patients with microscopic recognized T4 disease are excluded.
[b] Three N3 are included.

Table 3
Parietal pleura (PP) and muscle and rib (MR) invasion and N involvement

Study	PP+MR	Parietal Pleura Involvement			Muscle and Rib Involvement		
		N0	N1	N2	N0	N1	N2
Riquet et al[3]	44+81	21 (47.7%)	6 (13.6%)	17 (38.7%)	56 (69.1%)	7 (8.6%)	18 (22.3%)
Akay et al[11]	29+56	20 (69%)	5 (17.2%)	4 (13.8%)	44 (78.6%)	7 (12.5%)	5 (8.9%)
Doddoli et al[13]	138+171	91 (65.9%)	16 (11.6%)	31 (22.5%)	121 (70.8%)	16 (9.3%)	3 (19.9%)
Lin et al[14]	11+31	6 (54.5%)	5 (45.5%)		22 (71%)	9 (29%)	

Differences are not significant.

nontumoral pathologies such as infections (eg, tuberculosis, actinomycosis, hydatid cyst) may mimic T3 tumors with CW invasion, or the primary-secondary CW tumors with pulmonary invasion (although not as common as opposite state) as well, a preoperative diagnosis might totally change the treatment. The choice of approach will be influenced by lesion location and symptoms and in these tumors (peripheral), transthoracic aspiration biopsy under guidance of CT scan or US seems to be the procedure of choice. Fiberoptic bronchoscopy is usually nondiagnostic. Preoperative diagnosis is also necessary for considering the proper time of the adjuvant therapies.

NEOADJUVANT THERAPY

Neoadjuvant therapy, including chemotherapy and radiation therapy, may be helpful, as reported in patients with Pancoast tumors (T4).[2,29] However, this approach has not been tested in patients who have tumor invading the CW (T3).[2,25] Potential benefits are downstaging the tumor, decreasing the risk of tumor spillage during operation, allowing doubtful resectable tumors to be resected, and decreasing the rate of R1 and close margins, even if up to now this has not been demonstrated.[2] Chemotherapy has been tested in Stage IIIA and Stage B NSCLC, but mainly because of the N2 involvement and the T3N2 subgroup has not been targeted specifically. It should be advisable to include patients with pT3N2 in neoadjuvant treatment protocol trials and consider their results before definitely denying them a surgical chance of cure.

ADJUVANT THERAPY

Patterson and colleagues[30] reported in 1982 a 56% survival rate for patients who received radiation therapy versus a rate of 30% for those who did not, but it was not statistically significant. Facciolo and colleagues[7] observed a 74.1% survival

rate following radiation therapy versus a46.7% rate without radiation, a significant difference in univariate analysis that was not confirmed in multivariate analysis. Inversely, Doddoli and colleagues[13] did not observe any survival differences in univariate analysis between N0 and N1+N2 subgroups, whereas multivariate analysis demonstrated adjuvant therapy to significantly improve the prognosis in N1+N2 patients. Although suggested to be beneficial, adjuvant therapy has not yet significantly demonstrated its efficacy in several other studies.[3,6,8,10,14,17] Such results may simply reflect patient selection, patients with advanced tumors being more likely to be treated by radiation therapy. The issue remains unresolved, but radiation therapy does not seem to prevent local recurrence, which raises the question of reserving its use for highly selected patients or in the case of local recurrence. After nonradical resection or after extrapleural lobectomy for tumors infiltrating only the parietal pleura (with doubtful radicality), postoperative radiation therapy could be considered, but there is no evidence proving its benefit.

SUMMARY

En bloc CW and lung resection is not any more a surgical challenge, but surgical efficiency is still limited by the risk of incompletely resected tumor and the mediastinal LN involvement. The new challenge is thus to recognize new treatment modalities, including chemotherapy and radiation therapy innovations, likely to increase the chances of performing a complete resection and of better controlling the consequences of LN involvement.

REFERENCES

1. Coleman FP. Primary carcinoma of the lung with invasion of the ribs. Ann Surg 1947;126:156–68.
2. Stoelben E, Ludwig C. Chest wall resection for lung cancer: indications and techniques. Eur J Cardiothorac Surg 2009;35:450–6.

3. Riquet M, Lang-Lazdunski L, Le Pimpec Barthes F, et al. Characteristics and prognosis of resected T3 non-small cell lung cancer. Ann Thorac Surg 2002; 73:253–8.

4. Mountain CF. Revisions in the international system for staging lung cancer. Chest 1997;111:1710–7.

5. Edge SB, Byrd DR, Compton CC, et al. Lung. In: Edge SB, Byrd DR, Compton CC, et al, editors. AJCC cancer staging hand book. From the AJCC cancer staging manual. 7th edition. Chicago: Springer; 2010. p. 299–323.

6. Chapelier A, Fadel E, Macchiarini P, et al. Factors affecting long-term survival after en-bloc resection of lung cancer invading the chest wall. Eur J Cardiothorac Surg 2000;18:513–8.

7. Facciolo F, Cardillo G, Lopergolo M, et al. Chest wall invasion in non-small cell lung carcinoma: a rationale for en bloc resection. J Thorac Cardiovasc Surg 2001;121:649–56.

8. Magdeleinat P, Alifano M, Benbrahem C, et al. Surgical treatment of lung cancer invading the chest wall: results and prognostic factors. Ann Thorac Surg 2001;71:1094–9.

9. Elia S, Griffo S, Gentile M. Surgical treatment of lung cancer invading chest wall: a retrospective analysis of 110 patients. Eur J Cardiothorac Surg 2001;20: 356–60.

10. Burkhart H, Allen MS, Nichols FC III, et al. Results of en bloc resection for bronchogenic carcinoma with chest wall invasion. J Thorac Cardiovasc Surg 2002;123:670–5.

11. Akay H, Cangir AK, Kutlay H, et al. Surgical treatment of peripheral lung cancer adherent to the parietal pleura. Eur J Cardiothorac Surg 2002;22:615–20.

12. Matsuoka H, Nishio W, Okada M, et al. Resection of chest wall invasion in patients with non-small cell lung cancer. Eur J Cardiothorac Surg 2004;26: 1200–4.

13. Doddoli C, D'Journo B, Le Pimpec Barthes F, et al. Lung cancer invading the chest wall: a plea for en-bloc resection but the need for new treatment strategies. Ann Thorac Surg 2005;80:2032–40.

14. Lin YT, Hsu HS, Huang CS, et al. En bloc resection for lung cancer with chest wall invasion. J Chin Med Assoc 2006;69:157–61.

15. Martin-Ucar AE, Nicum R, Oey I, et al. En-bloc chest wall and lung resection for non-small cell lung cancer. Predictors of 60-day non-cancer related mortality. Eur J Cardiothorac Surg 2003;23:859–64.

16. Mineo TC, Ambrogi V, Pompeo E, et al. Immunohistochemistry-detected microscopic tumor spread affects outcome in en-bloc resection for T3-chest wall lung cancer. Eur J Cardiothorac Surg 2007;31: 1120–4.

17. Kawagushi K, Mori S, Usami N, et al. Preoperative evaluation of the depth of chest wall invasion and the extent of combined resections in lung cancer patients. Lung Cancer 2009;64:41–4.

18. DiPerna CA, Wood DE. Surgical management of T3 and T4 lung cancer. Clin Cancer Res 2005;11: 5038s–44s.

19. Mut M, Schiff D, Shaffrey ME. Metastasis to nervous system: spinal epidural and intramedullary metastases. J Neurooncol 2005;75:43–56.

20. Ratto GB, Piacenza G, Frola C, et al. Chest wall involvement by lung cancer: computed tomographic detection and results of operation. Ann Thorac Surg 1991;51:182–8.

21. Rendina EA, Bognolo DA, Mineo TC, et al. Computed tomography for the evaluation of intrathoracic invasion by lung cancer. J Thorac Cardiovasc Surg 1987;94:57–63.

22. Akata S, Kajiwara N, Park J, et al. Evaluation of chest wall invasion by lung cancer using respiratory dynamic MRI. J Med Imaging Radiat Oncol 2008; 52:36–9.

23. Bandi V, Lunn W, Ernst A, et al. Ultrasound vs CT in detecting chest wall invasion by tumor. Chest 2008; 133:881–6.

24. Suzuki N, Saitoh T, Kitamura S. Tumour invasion of the chest wall in lung cancer: diagnosis with US. Radiology 1993;187:39–42.

25. Allen MS. Chest wall resection and reconstruction for lung cancer. Thorac Surg Clin 2004;14:211–6.

26. Shamji MF, Maziak DF, Shamji FM, et al. Circulation of the spinal cord: an important consideration for thoracic surgeons. Ann Thorac Surg 2003;76: 315–21.

27. Satoh Y, Ishikawa Y, Inamura K, et al. Classification of parietal pleural invasion at adhesion sites with surgical specimens of lung cancer and implications for prognosis. Virchows Arch 2005;447:984–9.

28. Lardinois D, Müller M, Furrer M, et al. Functional assessment of chest wall integrity after methylmethacrylate reconstruction. Ann Thorac Surg 2000; 69:919–23.

29. Rusch VW, Parekh KR, Leon L, et al. Factors determining outcome after surgical resection of T3 and T4 lung cancers of the superior sulcus. J Thorac Cardiovasc Surg 2000;119:1147–53.

30. Patterson GA, Ilves R, Ginsberg RJ, et al. The value of adjuvant radiotherapy in pulmonary and chest wall resection for bronchogenic carcinoma. Ann Thorac Surg 1982;34:692–7.

Resection and Reconstruction for Primary Sternal Tumors

Alain Chapelier, MD, PhD[a,b],*

KEYWORDS

- Primary malignant sternal tumor
- Radiation-induced sarcoma • Radical resection
- Sternal reconstruction

Primary sternal tumors are uncommon: benign lesions are very rare and most sternal tumors are malignant, mostly sarcomas, arising either from the bone or soft tissues of the sternum.[1-3] Radical resection can offer a definitive cure of primary malignant sternal tumors (PMST), but the surgical management may be difficult because of the local aggressiveness of these tumors and a high recurrence rate. Improvement of reconstruction techniques with musculocutaneous flaps have made coverage of wide sternal defects reliable, especially after extensive skin excision.

DIAGNOSIS

The diagnosis of a sternal tumor is usually made clinically, on the basis of a palpable mass with or without pain in the sternal region. The tumor may be asymptomatic and only detected on imaging documents. The precise location of the tumor and the extent of sternal and chest wall involvement are determined by CT scan and MRI with sagittal views (**Fig. 1**). The diagnosis must be subsequently confirmed by a biopsy to distinguish primary from metastatic tumors and identify patients with a high-grade PMST whose primary treatment should be chemotherapy. An incisional biopsy is preferable to a needle biopsy for an accurate tissue diagnosis.[4]

Histology

PMST are mostly sarcomas, including several histologic types depicted in **Box 1**. Chondrosarcoma is the most frequent PMST. Histologic grading of soft tissue sarcomas is stated according to the international system.[5] Patients having received radiotherapy for breast cancer and Hodgkin disease are at long-term risk for development of a radiation-induced sarcoma (RIS) of the sternum. The median interval between the onset of radiotherapy and the occurrence of a RIS is around 14 years, and can be up to 25 years, and many of these tumors are high-grade sarcomas.[6-8]

PMST are rarely hematologic tumors (plasmacytomas and lymphomas) and may present as a localized sternal mass. A solitary plasmacytoma is eligible for sternal resection.[9] Treatment of primary sternal lymphoma is classically nonsurgical but resection can be proposed if the diagnosis is in doubt or in the case of persistent local disease after medical treatment.

All sternal tumors should be considered malignant until proven otherwise. Benign sternal tumors are very rare and consist of chondroma, bone cyst, fibrous dysplasia and hemangioma.[10] Furthermore, open biopsy may not distinguish between benign and malignant cartilaginous tumors and wide resection becomes necessary in questionable cases.

[a] Paris West University, 9 Bd d'Alambert, 78280 Guyancourt, France
[b] Department of Thoracic Surgery and Lung Transplantation, Hôpital Foch, 40 rue Worth, Suresnes, France
* Department of Thoracic Surgery and Lung Transplantation, Hôpital Foch, 40 rue Worth, Suresnes, France.
E-mail address: alain.chapelier@hopital-foch.org

Thorac Surg Clin 20 (2010) 529–534
doi:10.1016/j.thorsurg.2010.06.002
1547-4127/10/$ – see front matter © 2010 Elsevier Inc. All rights reserved.

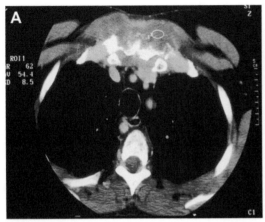
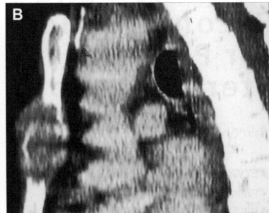

Fig. 1. (*A*) CT scan: massive invasion by a radiation induced fibrosarcoma. (*B*) Sagittal MRI scan: leiomyosarcoma of the sternal body.

PREOPERATIVE ASSESSMENT

The tumor extension and any infiltration of adjacent structures (lung, pericardium, brachiocephalic vein, and superior vena cava) are assessed by conventional axial CT scanning and MRI. PET CT scanning is mostly used to eliminate an extrathoracic metastatic lesion. Every patient is routinely evaluated with cardiopulmonary tests; a severe respiratory insufficiency should be a contra indication for an extensive sternal resection.

Box 1
Primary sternal tumors histologic types
Malignant
Sarcomas
Chondrosarcoma
Osteosarcoma
Fibrosarcoma
Malignant fibrous histiocytoma
Leiomyosarcoma
Angiosarcoma
Ewing sarcoma
Undifferentiated
Hematologic diseases
Plasmacytoma
Hodgkin lymphoma
Benign
Chondroma
Fibrous dysplasia
Bone cysts
Hemangioma

The closure of wide sternal defects is planned by both the thoracic and plastic surgeons in difficult cases. Chemotherapy is advocated for patients with Ewing sarcomas and high-grade sarcomas of the sternum followed by sternal resection.

OPERATIVE PROCEDURE
Resection

Wide excision remains the key to success for local control of PMST.

The first step is the skin excision. When the skin and overlying soft tissues are not involved, a vertical elliptical incision encompassing the biopsy site is done. The skin excision must be large in cases of ulceration, previous scars, and if the tumor involves subcutaneous tissues. RIS of the sternum frequently requires a wide cutaneous excision, including previously irradiated surrounding tissues with a margin of at least 2 cm of macroscopically tissues.

Sternal resection must include wide resection of the affected part of the sternum; clear margins of at least 3 cm are advocated to minimize the risk of local recurrence.[11] Resection is started over the costal margins, sparing the unaffected lateral part of the pectoralis major (PM) muscles, and the pleural space is opened on both sides. A total sternectomy, including the internal third of clavicles, is undertaken for tumors involving both parts of the bone, for large tumors of the mid sternum, and in the case of an Ewing sarcoma. A subtotal sternectomy is performed, sparing the uppermost 2 cm of the manubrium and clavicles in the case of tumors invading the sternal body. A partial sternectomy is performed for tumors limited to the manubrium or the lower part of the sternum. Resection has to be extended to the adjacent anterior chest wall if invaded by the tumor. Tumor extension into the chest cavity is evaluated. Lung and involved mediastinal structures have to be excised en bloc. Invasion of brachiocephalic veins is managed by ligation and excision; involvement of the superior vena cava may require resection and polytetrafluoroethylene (PTFE) revascularization. After sternal resection, a chest tube is placed in each pleural cavity.

Sternal Reconstruction

The reconstruction must afford enough stability and adequate airtight closure.

Chest wall stability

Skeletal reconstruction is recommended for protective and cosmetic reasons and to stabilize the chest wall. Chest wall stability after a wide sternectomy can be obtained with different prosthetic materials such as polyglactin mesh (Ethnor Inc, Summerville, NJ, USA), Marlex mesh (Bard Inc, Murray Hill, NJ, USA), or PTFE patch (W.L. Gore & Assoc, Flagstaff, AZ, USA). The respective advantages of each material have already been outlined.[12] Marlex mesh, offers a good incorporation into the tissues but, in the case of contamination, its removal is laborious. The use of a 2 mm thick, soft tissue PTFE patch, which can be easily fixed under tension to the edges of the sternal defect with interrupted nonabsorbable sutures, is now advocated by many surgeons. It provides a watertight closure and the patch is easily visible on the CT scan in the follow-up so that a local recurrence is more easily detected.[13,14]

Usually, an adequate skeletal stability without rigid reconstruction is obtained with a prosthetic patch alone if a significant part of the sternum is preserved (**Fig. 2**). After a total or subtotal sternectomy, a rigid prosthetic replacement is recommended to avoid flail chest and to minimize the risk of respiratory complications. Autogenous tissues, such as rib and bone grafts, have been proposed for sternal reconstruction with minimal success. Until recently, the methylmethacrylate has been frequently used to reconstruct wide sternal defects, usually spread between two layers of Marlex mesh or spread on a PTFE patch.[15,16] If dislocation of the prosthesis has been observed, the major pitfall of reconstruction with methylmethacrylate is infection. A high incidence of infection has been reported in recent large series,[3,17] requiring complete removal of the composite infected material. Consequently, the risks of infection should be balanced against the functional and protective benefits of rigid prosthetic sternal reconstruction. Because of the risks of dislocation and wound infection, metallic materials are not recommended for chest wall reconstruction for tumors. However, interest has been renewed by the use of moldable titanium bars and rib clips (Strasbourg Thoracic Osteosyntheses System STRATOS; MedXpert GmbH, Heitersheim, Germany) for chest wall deformities reconstruction, which has been recently extended for tumors.[18,19] This system offers numerous advantages: high tissue compatibility, resistance to infection and improved CT scan and MRI. In our recent 5 years experience of ten sternectomies for primary tumors, reconstruction with PTFE patch was reinforced by STRATOS bars and clips in four cases of total or subtotal sternectomy with excellent results (**Fig. 3**).

Soft tissue coverage

Soft tissue coverage is the essential step of sternal reconstruction and can be obtained with muscle or musculocutaneous flaps.[20] PM muscles are the most frequently selected muscles transferred to the sternal defect with skin advancement on the

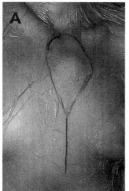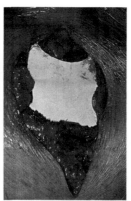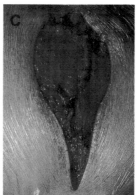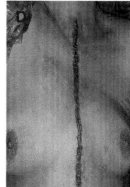

Fig. 2. Leiomyosarcoma of the manubrium. (*A*) Clinical presentation. (*B*) PTFE 2 mm patch after a partial sternectomy. (*C*) Reconstruction with PM muscles. (*D*) Final result.

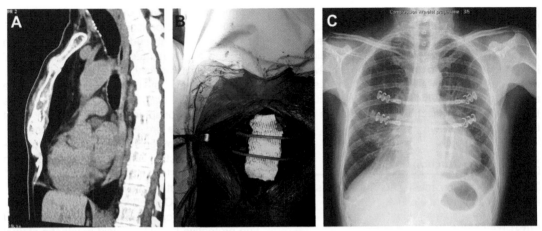

Fig. 3. Chondrosarcoma of the sternal body. (*A*) CT scan. (*B*) Reconstruction reinforced by STRATOS bars after a subtotal sternectomy sparing the uppermost of the manubrium. (*C*) Postoperative radiograph.

front line. If necessary, section of the humeral insertion can afford a better rotation with no tension on the vascular pedicle. After a wide skin and subcutaneous excision, reconstruction of sternal and soft tissue defects can be achieved by the combined efforts of the thoracic and plastic surgeons. Musculocutaneous flaps afford an airtight closure and a well vascularized reliable sternal reconstruction (**Fig. 4**). A PM musculocutaneous flap can be done in men; it can also be used bilaterally in the case of a very large sternal defect extended to the neck.[13]

A latissimus dorsi (LD) musculocutaneous flap is usually employed with skin closure of the donor site.[21,22] In some cases of PMST in women, it is possible to preserve the LD flap as previously done. A breast flap may also be an acceptable option in an elderly woman who had undergone

prior mastectomy. Free flaps (LD, rectus abdominis) are now a reliable option if no regional musculocutaneous flap is available. Suction drains have to be placed in dead spaces at the end of the operation.

An omentoplasty can be interposed in some difficult cases, such as resection in irradiated fields, and for recurrent tumors (**Table 1**).[23]

POSTOPERATIVE COURSE
Local Complications

The occurrence of a seroma is frequent after reconstruction with PTFE, and it usually resorbs in a few weeks. In the case of large seroma, aspiration will be done under strict aseptic conditions. Wound infection is a major concern occurring in the immediate postoperative period requiring

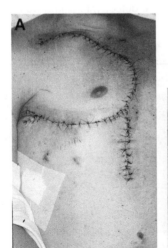
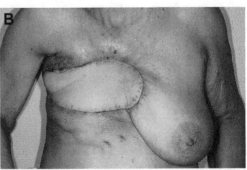

Fig. 4. Soft tissue reconstruction with musculocutaneous flaps. (*A*) Pectoralis major. (*B*) Latissimus dorsi.

Table 1
Sternal reconstruction

Prosthetic Material	Soft Tissue Coverage
Polyglactin mesh Marlex mesh PTFE 2 mm patch	PM translation with skin advancement Breast flap

Rigid reinforcement
  Methylmethacrylate
  STRATOS[a] system
	Musculocutaneous
	  flap
	PM unilateral
	  LD
	PM bilateral
	Free flap (LD,
	  Rectus Abdominis)

	Associated omentoplasty

[a] STRATOS, MedXpert GmbH, Heitersheim, Germany.

operative debridement or being delayed after several weeks or months, with a risk of prosthesis contamination. In the case of infection with rigid reconstruction with methylmethacrylate, complete removal of the prosthetic infected material is needed. With a PTFE patch alone, a conservative treatment may be possible. However, removal of the infected patch can be required and is easily done if necessary; the fibrous tissues usually yields enough stability of the chest wall at that time.

Flap-related complications are rare; in the case of flap loss another flap can be done, but omentoplasty is an alternative option.

Respiratory Complications

Respiratory complications include pneumonia that can be associated with septicemia and respiratory failure, which may require a prolonged ventilatory support and a tracheostomy. Respiratory complications are the main cause of mortality.[3,17]

The role of adjuvant chemotherapy after complete resection of a PMST is still debated, yet advocated, for patients based on the high grading of the tumor and with respect to a primary medical treatment. CT scan at 3 and 6 months, 1 year, and each year thereafter for at least 5 years are recommended to detect a local recurrence and identify pulmonary metastases in the follow-up.

Recurrence

In selected patients with limited local recurrence or single metastasis, a repeat resection is possible.

Local recurrence
Local recurrences can be either a bony recurrence that may require a completion sternectomy or

a limited, soft tissue recurrence treated by a repeat resection. This highlights the importance of wide excision of skin and soft tissue, especially in the case of RIS of the sternum where the interpretation of frozen sections is particularly difficult.

Systemic recurrence
Lung metastases can be resected if single or few. The benefit of sternal resection for a solitary plasmacytoma is jeopardized by the frequent development of multiple myeloma in the follow-up.[1,3]

Survival
The overall 5-year survival after radical sternal resection and reconstruction for PMST was 66% in our previous series.[3] Survival in completely resected patients is related to the histologic grade of sarcomas as previously reported by several authors: high-grade tumors are an adverse factor for long-term survival.[3,24] The presence of pulmonary metastases at initial presentation and the occurrence of recurrence in the follow-up are also adverse survival predictors.[25]

SUMMARY

Radical resection of PMST and satisfactory reconstruction of wide sternal defects can be safely performed. Whereas reconstruction after a partial sternectomy is usually done with a PTFE patch and PM transposition with skin advancement, a rigid reinforcement of the sternum can now be achieved with titanium bars and clips after a total sternectomy.

Large sternal defects are safely reconstructed with a musculocutaneous flap, especially in the case of radiation-induced sarcomas. The completeness of the resection and the histologic grade of the tumors are the strongest survival predictors.

REFERENCES

1. Martini N, Huvos AG, Burt ME, et al. Predictors of survival in malignant tumors of the sternum. J Thorac Cardiovasc Surg 1996;111:96–106.
2. Incarbone M, Nava M, Lequaglie C, et al. Sternal resection for primary or secondary tumors. J Thorac Cardiovasc Surg 1997;114:93–9.
3. Chapelier A, Missana MC, Couturaud B, et al. Sternal resection and reconstruction for primary tumors. Ann Thorac Surg 2004;77:1001–7.
4. Soysal O, Walsh GL, Nesbitt JC, et al. Resection of sternal tumors: extent, reconstruction, and survival. Ann Thorac Surg 1995;60:1353–8.
5. Coindre JM, Trojani M, Contesso G, et al. Reproducibility of a histopathologic grading system for adult soft tissue sarcoma. Cancer 1986;58:306–9.

6. Souba WW, Mc Kenna RJ, Meis J, et al. Radiation-induced sarcomas of the chest wall. Cancer 1986; 57:610–5.

7. Brady MS, Garfein CF, Petrek JA, et al. Post-treatment sarcoma in breast cancer patients. Ann Surg Oncol 1994;1:66–72.

8. Chapelier A, Bacha E, De Montpreville VT, et al. Radical resection of radiation-induced sarcoma of the chest-wall: report of 15 cases. Ann Thorac Surg 1997;63:214–9.

9. Burt M, Karpeh M, Ukoha O, et al. Medical tumors of the chest wall. Solitary plasmacytoma and Ewing's sarcoma. J Thorac Cardiovasc Surg 1993;105: 89–96.

10. Onat S, Ulku R, Avci A, et al. Hemangioma of the sternum. Ann Thorac Surg 2008;86:1974–6.

11. King RM, Pairolero PC, Trastek VF, et al. Primary chest wall tumors: factors affecting survival. Ann Thorac Surg 1986;41:597–601.

12. McCormack PM. Use of prosthetic materials in chest-wall reconstruction. Surg Clin North Am 1989;69:965–76.

13. Chapelier A, Macchiarini P, Rietjens M, et al. Chest wall reconstruction following resection of large primary malignant tumors. Eur J Cardiothorac Surg 1994;8:351–7.

14. Deschamps C, Tirnaksiz BM, Darbandi R, et al. Early and long-term results of prosthetic chest wall reconstruction. J Thorac Cardiovasc Surg 1999;117: 588–92.

15. Boyd AD, Shaw WW, McCarthy JG, et al. Immediate reconstruction of full thickness chest wall defects. Ann Thorac Surg 1980;32:337–46.

16. Lardinois D, Müller M, Furrer M, et al. Functional assessment of chest wall integrity after methylmethacrylate reconstruction. Ann Thorac Surg 2000;69:919–23.

17. Weyant MJ, Bains MS, Venkatraman E, et al. Results of chest wall resection and reconstruction with and without rigid prosthesis. Ann Thorac Surg 2006;81: 279–85.

18. Coonar AS, Qureshi N, Smith I, et al. A novel titanium rib bridge system for chest wall reconstruction. Ann Thorac Surg 2009;87(5):e46–8.

19. Gonfiotti A, Santini PF, Campanacci D, et al. Use of moldable titanium bars and rib clips for total sternal replacement: a new composite technique. J Thorac Cardiovasc Surg 2009;138:1248–50.

20. Arnold PG, Pairolero PC. Use of pectoralis major muscle flap to repair defects of the anterior chest wall. Plast Reconstr Surg 1979;63:205–13.

21. Moelleken BR, Mathes SA, Chang N. Latissimus dorsi muscle musculocutaneous flap in chest wall reconstruction. Surg Clin North Am 1989;69: 977–90.

22. Rocco G, Scognamiglio F, Fazioli F, et al. V-Y latissimus dorsi flap for coverage of anterior chest wall defects after resection of recurrent chest wall chondrosarcoma. J Thorac Cardiovasc Surg 2009;138: 1242–3.

23. Mansour KA, Anderson TM, Hester TR. Sternal resection and reconstruction. Ann Thorac Surg 1993;55:838–43.

24. Burt M, Fulton M, Wessner-Dunlap S, et al. Primary bony and cartilaginous sarcomas of chest wall; results of therapy. Ann Thorac Surg 1992;54: 226–32.

25. McAfee MK, Pairolero PC, Bergstralh EJ, et al. Chondrosarcoma of the chest wall; factors affecting survival. Ann Thorac Surg 1985;40:535–41.

Outcomes of Surgery for Chest Wall Sarcomas

Joe B. Putnam Jr, MD

KEYWORDS

• Sarcoma • Chest wall • Outcomes • Survival

Chest wall sarcomas, as other sarcomas, originate from tissues of mesenchymal origin. These uncommon tumors infrequently involve the bony thorax, soft tissues of the chest wall, or sternum.[1–4] The tumors grow by local extension until size or symptoms develop, although occasionally diagnosis is made when the size of the mass becomes noticeable, or symptoms occur such as pain or functional limitation, or when a painless mass occurs. In a recent experience of 51 patients who presented with primary sarcomas of the chest wall, the median age was 47 years and pain was the most common presenting symptom (n = 23) followed by an asymptomatic mass (n = 13).[1]

Sarcomas may arise from adjacent structures and may locally extend to the chest wall. These structures include the lung, the breast, radiation-associated sarcomas arising from previously irradiated areas of the chest wall (generally following many years after breast cancer and adjuvant radiotherapy), mediastinum, or diaphragm. Metastatic lesions to the chest wall can also occur.[5,6]

Wide local excision with negative margins and reconstruction of the defect after primary tumor excision are needed to optimize function and appearance.[7] A multispecialty surgical team complements the multidisciplinary treatment planning team. This integrated multidisciplinary management plan should include evaluation by the thoracic surgeon, medical oncologist, and radiation oncologist. A reconstructive surgeon may assist with complex muscle flaps (including free tissue transfer), or reconstruction of tissues that are heavily radiated. Local recurrence is uncommon after complete resection, and if needed, re-resection may be considered. Local extirpation remains the most effective therapy, albeit local recurrence can occur. Nevertheless, survival is limited by distant metastases.

PATIENT SELECTION

Patients with primary chest wall sarcomas should be selected for resection based on standard oncologic criteria. Patients should be evaluated for the extent of their disease and if an operation can be tolerated safely. General oncologic principles apply, including absence of uncontrolled extrathoracic disease and physiologic fitness for general anesthesia and the proposed resection. Evaluation of diaphragmatic function with fluoroscopy to examine bilateral diaphragm excursion or paradoxic movement during inspiration (the "sniff test") may be helpful in planning extent of operation along with the critical need to preserve the single remaining phrenic nerve. Redo operations from incomplete initial operation create a more complex situation for complete resection with negative margins. Division of the latissimus dorsi muscle from previous thoracotomy may have occurred and will affect reconstruction options. Previous abdominal operations should be reviewed. Patients with a prior coronary artery bypass operation, or tumors involving this previous operative field, may require a more complex resection to preserve the vascular grafts and cardiac function.

DIAGNOSIS

Diagnosis entails a careful evaluation of the patient with history and physical examination, plain chest radiography, and computed tomography of the

No conflicts of interest.

Department of Thoracic Surgery, Vanderbilt University Medical Center, 1313 21st Avenue South, 609 Oxford House, Nashville, TN 37232-4682, USA

E-mail address: bill.putnam@vanderbilt.edu

Thorac Surg Clin 20 (2010) 535–542
doi:10.1016/j.thorsurg.2010.07.005

chest.[8,9] Sarcomas tend to metastasize to the lungs and synchronous pulmonary metastases are associated with poorer prognosis. Magnetic resonance imaging can assist in the evaluation of the relationship of the tumor to the intrathoracic structures and potentially the interactions at the tumor–normal tissue interface. In addition, a fluorodeoxyglucose positron emission tomography (FDG PET) scan could be used to evaluate metabolic activity, bony destruction, and potential sites of metastases.

Fine-needle or core-needle biopsy may provide a diagnosis before treatment, thus avoiding an incisional biopsy. Incisional biopsies can contaminate the surrounding tissue necessitating a much larger resection and a significant chest wall defect. In these patients, the rate of malignancy can reach 50% to 80%; as a rule, these tumors require an en bloc resection. Open biopsy should be reserved only for those patients in whom repeat needle biopsy did not provide a definitive diagnosis. A preoperative consultation with the bone radiologist and selective use of fine-needle or trephine biopsies should be appropriate for diagnosis and interim planning.

TECHNIQUES OF RESECTION AND RECONSTRUCTION

Resection for local control of sarcomas is based on accurate diagnosis, complete extirpation of all disease with negative margins, and adequate reconstruction to maintain or improve physiologic function. The outcomes of resection have been evaluated by various centers with collected series. Because of the relative rarity of such tumors, treatment paradigms have been based on results of retrospective reviews. According to these series, both simple and complex resections can be accomplished safely. The general practice of thoracic surgeons is to offer patients with chest wall or sternal sarcomas a surgical option to provide long-term and disease-free survival.

The soft tissue flaps that are available to the thoracic and to the reconstructive surgeon are numerous.[10] In fact, all chest wall muscles can be rotated. Moreover, a free muscle flap can be implanted with microvascular anastomosis, providing an alternative if previous operations or radiotherapy have compromised muscle flap choices for reconstruction.

Sternal resection provides a more formidable challenge for both resection and reconstruction than simple chest wall surgical procedures.[11] Any portion of the sternum can be resected or the sternum may be resected in its entirety. Elective resection of the sternum requires rigid prosthetic reconstruction to stabilize the thoracic cage. Coverage of the prosthesis with adjacent musculature (pectoralis major muscle, latissimus dorsi, rectus abdominis) or other tissue (eg, omentum) is recommended.

A margin of 3 to 5 cm of normal tissue is needed for radical resection of primary chest wall sarcomas. A margin of one healthy rib superiorly and inferiorly is recommended.[12] Local extension from the chest wall sarcoma into other structures, such as lung, diaphragm, and pericardium, is not a contraindication to resection.[2] However, the thoracic surgeon must be confident that a complete resection can be accomplished and subsequent reconstruction performed safely to allow a functional recovery. Reportedly, en bloc resection can be performed with good results.[13]

Chondrosarcomas are most frequently encountered and complete resection with a negative margin is required.[14] Locally invasive tumors, such as desmoid or myxoid neoplasms, may not metastasize distantly but may recur locally. Should this occur, significant morbidity for subsequent operation may be noted, particularly if an inadequate resection was performed initially.

The entire tumor and involved soft tissue must be removed completely with negative margins, particularly in sternal tumors.[11,15] In patients with sternal tumors involving only a portion of the sternum, a complete sternectomy may not be required. Maintaining the integrity of the thoracic inlet (the junction of the clavicle, first rib, and upper [cephalad] half of the manubrium) may facilitate the patient's recovery and enhance recovery of pulmonary function. Alternatively, the sternum may remain stabilized with the lower half of the sternum remaining in position. Stabilization of the manubrium area with a prosthetic patch or a tailored composite Marlex-methylmethacrylate prosthesis is recommended. Frozen section analysis of margins in question should be performed based on the clinical findings and guide the extent of resection. In this setting, chest wall resection in children can be performed safely with good results.[16–23]

Only patients with large chest wall defects (roughly estimating an area larger than the patient's palm) would require stabilization with Marlex mesh.[10] Patients with resection of ribs 1, 2, 3, and 4 may not require any reconstruction because of the overlying scapula posteriorly and chest wall musculature (anterior and posterior). If the ribs are resected underneath the tip of the scapula, limited resection of the scapula (inferior 30%–50%) or prosthetic reconstruction of the inferior portion of the chest wall may be needed so as not to cause a "trapped scapula" with depression of the scapula into the thorax. Marlex mesh provides an excellent highly effective and cost-effective prostatic material. Ingrowth of fibroblasts assists in providing further stabilization of this material over time. A sandwich of 2 layers of Marlex prosthesis with an acrylic methylmethacrylate gel can be used for rigid reconstruction of portions of the chest wall. Other prosthetic materials include Prolene mesh or 2-mm thick or "thin" 1-mm Gore-Tex (polytetrafluoroethylene) soft tissue patch.[24] The Gore-Tex is impervious to fluid and may be considered for resections involving the diaphragm. Both Marlex mesh and Gore-Tex prostheses are effective for chest wall reconstruction.[25]

OUTCOMES OF CHEST WALL AND STERNAL RESECTION FOR PRIMARY SARCOMA

Chest wall resection and reconstruction can range from simple extirpation, without reconstruction, to a formidable operation requiring multispecialty surgical teams.[6,20,26–28] A detailed atlas describing the varieties of chest wall resection and reconstruction has been published.[29] The sequence of multispecialty care within the operating room is critical to the successful outcome for the patient. A thoracic surgical team and a plastic/reconstructive surgical team, both experienced in thoracic reconstruction, must plan preoperatively and implement surgical care intraoperatively to achieve optimal results.[30,31] The preoperative and physiologic status must be considered to optimize the postoperative care and in-hospital convalescence.

Prognostic factors that affect both recurrence and survival for primary chest wall sarcomas are similar to that of other primary tissue sarcomas, ie, tumor grade, presence of distant metastasis, or positive surgical margins.[32] "Benign" lesions may account for a significant number of primary chest-wall neoplasms in some series.[31] In this context, some locations are typical, such as chondromas arising at the costochondral junction or fibrous dysplasia in a posterior or lateral rib. Treatment of these tumors is by complete resection.

PRIMARY BONE SARCOMAS OF THE CHEST WALL

Chondrosarcoma is the most common primary chest wall malignancy.[4,33,34] It accounts for 30% to 50% of malignant neoplasms and 25% of all primary chest wall tumors.[35] Eighty percent of chondrosarcomas arise in the ribs and 20% arise in the sternum.[36] Most tumors are solitary and are present for months to years before presentation or diagnosis. The treatment of choice is wide local excision including ribs above and below the lesion. Ten-year survival rates are good (95%) after wide local excision.[37] In one recent series, 106 patients with chondrosarcoma of the rib or sternum were treated over 22 years (1980 to 2002). Of these, 97 patients were treated with curative intent. Wide local excision resulted in a 10-year survival of 92%. Factors associated with local recurrence included surgical margin and histologic grade.[14]

Ewing sarcoma is the most common primary chest wall malignancy in children[21,38,39] and consists of small, round cells with characteristics of a primitive neuroectodermal tumor (PNET).[40,41] About two-thirds of these tumors occur in children younger than 20 years.[38] Ewing sarcoma occurs in fewer than 25% of malignant chest wall lesions in adults. The differential diagnosis can include neuroblastoma, embryonal rhabdomyosarcoma, angiosarcoma, extraosseous Ewing sarcoma, or lymphoma. Ewing sarcoma and PNET are grouped together because of common neuroectodermal origins, and similar genetic translocations. The diagnosis and treatment are similar.[42] Early metastases to the lungs and bones occur. Pretreatment evaluation should include computed tomography of the chest and bone marrow aspiration. The radiographic appearance is characteristic "onion-peel" produced by a new bone periosteal formation. The diagnosis is made by needle biopsy. The entire marrow is considered to be at risk for malignant involvement. Generally, the entire involved rib must be removed. A partial rib resection above and below the lesion can also be of added value.

Postoperative radiation therapy can be given for local control. Neoadjuvant chemotherapy and delayed resection of chest wall Ewing sarcoma (PNET) increased the likelihood of an R0 complete tumor resection and avoided adjuvant radiotherapy.[43]

Osteogenic sarcoma has a bimodal distribution with occurrences in the second decade of life and again in the fourth decade of life. A biopsy is typically needed to provide treatment recommendations. A radiographic "sunburst" pattern of periosteal bone formation may be identified. Preoperative chemotherapy with doxorubicin, methotrexate, and cis-platinum may be considered. Preoperative chemotherapy before surgery provides for a biologic response and shrinkage of the tumor, minimizing the operation required, preventing tumor-resistant clones from developing, treating systemic metastasis present, and with normal blood supply preoperatively, optimal chemotherapeutic dispersion may be achieved. Radiation therapy after surgery is not generally performed.

Soft tissue sarcomas of the chest wall are uncommon.[44] These tumors often present as a painless, gradually enlarging mass. Some of these tumors are radiation associated. These tumors may spread for some considerable distance from the primary tumor and insinuate themselves along fascial planes or between muscle fibers. Chemotherapy may provide some advantage if the diagnosis is made before surgery with needle biopsy. Reducing the size of the tumor may make the operation more technically feasible, and increase potential for negative margins.[4,32,45,46]

Desmoid tumors may be difficult to distinguish from low-grade fibrosarcomas and may represent a spectrum of disease.[47] Of these tumors, 40% may occur in the chest wall and shoulder area. Desmoid tumors can be of any size and consist of well-differentiated fibroblasts and collagen that lack encapsulation. These physical findings create problems in determining the extent of resection. Resection or enucleation of the tumor may be valuable options.[47] Although this tumor grows slowly and does not metastasize, local control can be an issue in many patients. As a consequence, these tumors should be excised with at least 4-cm margins; however, larger resection margins may be helpful, as these tumors spread along fascial planes. Although only about half of patients with positive resection margins recur, these tumors are sensitive to high-dose radiation therapy, which may be helpful for local control after resection. Tamoxifen has been used with some success in treating these tumors.[48]

In one series,[32] malignant fibrous histiocytoma (MFH) was the most common soft tissue chest wall tumor. MFH has a high rate of local recurrence and distal metastases,[49] and wide local excision is the recommended treatment.

Rhabdomyosarcoma in its 3 subtypes (ie, alveolar, embryonal, and pleomorphic), extraosseous Ewing sarcoma, and undifferentiated sarcomas are responsive to chemotherapy. Multidisciplinary treatment should include induction chemotherapy, wide local excision, and postoperative chemotherapy. Resection is performed when chemotherapy response has stabilized. Local radiation can be used for positive margins or if surgical resection is not feasible.

Solitary plasmacytomas may arise in bone and may account for 10% to 30% of primary chest wall malignancies.[50] These tumors are more common in men (mean age 60) and located in the ribs. Localized plasmacytoma must be confirmed by excluding other locations (bone marrow aspiration, radiographic bone survey, and immunoelectrophoresis of the serum and urine). Radiation therapy of 50 to 60 Gy may be successful for local control. Surgery may be required if the lesion is not responsive. Systemic chemotherapy should be considered in the event of disease progression.[6]

RESULTS OF THERAPY— SINGLE-INSTITUTION STUDIES

In one series, 51 patients were treated over a 10-year period with no mortality and a 94% R0 resection rate.[1] Forty patients were initially treated at the primary institution, whereas 11 patients were treated after unsuccessful surgical excision elsewhere. Pain and an expanding mass were the most common presenting symptoms. Neoplasms were located in the ribs (n = 36), sternum (n = 11), and in the rib with associated invasion into the vertebral body (n = 4). Histotypes included chondrosarcoma (15), MFH (9), osteogenic sarcoma (4), Ewing sarcoma (3), desmoid tumor (7), or others (13). Approximately half of all patients received some induction therapy (26/51 patients), with 22 patients receiving chemotherapy alone. A complete sternectomy was performed in 6 of 11 patients with sternal tumors; 4 patients had vertebral body resections. Reconstruction was accomplished with a prosthetic mesh alone in 16 of 51 patients. More complex rigid prostheses consisting of a mesh with methylmethacrylate was used in 18 of 51 patients. Furthermore, 24 patients had muscle flap reconstruction. In 47 of 51 patients an R0 resection status was achieved. In 12 patients, overall morbidity was reported as mild to moderate. Adjuvant therapy consisted of chemotherapy alone (n = 9) or chemoradiotherapy (n = 4). With an average follow-up of 44.7 months, the 5-year survival was 64% (initial referral, 61.3%; secondary referral, 72.7%). The authors recommended an aggressive multidisciplinary approach to these primary sarcomas of the chest wall given the excellent outcomes and prolonged 5-year survival. Factors associated with improved 5-year survival included tumor location in the sternum, tumor size smaller than 500 cm^3, desmoid tumor or chondrosarcoma, and negative margins. Factors associated with overall recurrence-free 5-year survival included tumor location in the sternum, desmoid tumor, or chondrosarcoma, and use of perioperative chemotherapy, radiation therapy, or both.

In one Japanese study, more than 70% of patients had undergone previous excision. Wide local excision was subsequently accomplished. Despite this previous excision, the overall 5-year survival was 88.5%.[51]

Chemotherapy regimens have included doxorubicin, cisplatin, high-dose methotrexate, and standard and high-dose ifosfamide. Chemotherapy may reduce the size of the tumor to increase the likelihood of negative margins and to treat micrometastases. Furthermore, chemotherapy can identify patients who have a biologic response to such treatment.

Combined thoracic surgery and neurosurgery resections are not commonly performed; however, experienced teams can achieve excellent results.[52] Resection of ribs and vertebral body can be accomplished with stabilization of the thoracic column with Harrington rods and vertebral replacement or reconstruction. Thoracic stabilization and coverage by the reconstructive surgeons is frequently required.[53]

SPECIAL CIRCUMSTANCES

A significant number of chest wall tumors are secondary rather than primary neoplasms. In one series, one-third of chest wall resections were performed for metastatic lesions. In patients with metastatic sarcomas to the chest wall, response to chemotherapy and isolated site of recurrence appeared to be favorable prognostic factors.[7]

Radiation-associated sarcomas may occur years after therapeutic radiation therapy for breast or thoracic neoplasms.[54–58] In one series, 8 patients had radiation-associated sarcomas from radiation for Hodgkin lymphoma, breast cancer, lung cancer, and Wilms tumor. The sarcomas occurred in the radiation fields; the mean time interval was 9 years and the average radiation dose was 48 Gy. These patients should be treated with wide local excision. Complete resection of high-grade sarcomas produced a 5-year survival of approximately 56% versus a 40-month survival of 20% with radiation-induced sarcomas ($P = .11$).[1] These patients should be offered treatment identical to that of patients with primary tumors. Another recent study noted that radiation-associated soft tissue sarcomas were most commonly MFH and had a disease-specific survival of 44% compared with a matched cohort of other MFH patients ($P = .07$).[59] Factors associated with poorer survival in patients with radiation-associated sarcomas were size larger than 5 cm, margin positivity, and histologic type. In another 67 patients, an R0 resection was achieved in 75% of patients. Overall, 5-year survival was 45%, whereas the local relapse rate was 65%.[58]

Vertebral body or transverse processes may become involved with sarcoma of the chest wall, which extend posteriorly to involve the transverse process or lateral vertebral body. Both metastases to the vertebral body and primary tumors of the vertebral body can occur. Satisfactory results have been obtained using anterior vertebral body resection, reconstruction, and stabilization. In one series of 72 patients with metastatic spinal tumors treated by transthoracic vertebrectomy, melanoma or sarcoma occurred in 10. Back pain was the most common symptom (90%) and lower extremity weakness (64%) also occurred. Using a 2-team approach with thoracic surgery and neurosurgery, patients underwent transthoracic vertebrectomy, decompression, reconstruction with methylmethacrylate, and anterior fixation with locking plate and screw constructs. Supplemental posterior instrumentation with rods was required in some patients. Pain was significantly reduced after surgery and neurologic dysfunction was also improved significantly. Thirty-day mortality rate was 3% and the 1-year survival rate of all 72 patients was 62%. Transthoracic vertebrectomy and spinal stabilization improved quality of life in these patients by improving or restoring ambulation and by reducing spinal pain.[52]

Great vessel involvement by primary chest wall or sternal sarcomas is unusual. Although wide local excision is required, if the great vessels or the heart are involved with tumor, the surgeon must make a decision as to whether the extent of the tumor warrants resection and reconstruction of the involved vessels, or if an incomplete resection (with positive margins) should be performed given that the early risks of resection are greater than the early risks of a positive margins.[60]

OTHER CHEST WALL SARCOMA INVOLVEMENT

Patients with tumors involving the lateral aspect of the shoulder girdle, upper humerus, or distal clavicle may require forequarter amputation.[61] On occasion, this operation may be extended because of sarcomatous involvement of the first, second, or third ribs. A 2-team approach with general surgery and thoracic surgery is used. Once local resection of the primary tumor and, as well, resection of the deep chest wall margin with wide local excision is performed, reconstruction with a Vicryl mesh or a Marlex mesh may be used to provide for stabilization of this area. With the arm and shoulder blade and shoulder girdle removed, compression of the underlying lung may occur. Stabilization of this area may assist in postoperative respiratory function.

Local recurrence of chest wall sarcomas portends an ominous prognosis. As the original operation was performed with wide local excision to alleviate the potential for local recurrence, local recurrence may suggest a much more aggressive tumor than previously recognized. If the tumor is solitary and, after appropriate staging, only a local recurrence is found, then re-resection can be attempted. Before resection, chemotherapy could be considered. Again, resection and reconstruction must be performed with wide local excisions.[62]

STERNAL SARCOMAS

Resection and reconstruction of the sternum uses the same principle as that of chest wall resection.[5,15,28] In one series of 52 patients with sternal tumors treated over 13 years, malignant tumors were found in 20 patients. Total sternectomy was performed in only a minority of patients (n = 5). Subtotal sternectomy was performed in 19 patients and partial resection, defined as less than 50% of the sternum, was performed in 28 patients. Prosthetic material and/or flap coverage was used in 83% of patients. Five-year survival for all patients was 46%. Of the 20 primary malignant tumors, 19 were sarcomas, namely chondrosarcoma (7 patients); osteogenic sarcoma (3); Askin tumor (2); soft tissue sarcoma not otherwise specified (3); and liposarcoma, leiomyosarcoma, rhabdomyosarcoma, and angiosarcoma (1 patient each). In addition, desmoid tumors were found in 4 patients.[63]

In another series of 30 patients treated with sternectomy, 13 patients had primary sternal sarcoma, including chondrosarcoma (6 patients), osteosarcoma (5), and others (2). In most patients, 5-cm margins were achieved. The technique of reconstruction included muscle flap alone in 13 patients, muscle flap and mesh in 9 patients, muscle flap and rigid prosthesis (Marlex methylmethacrylate) in 7 patients, or other in 1 patient. Five-year actuarial survival after primary sternal sarcoma tumor resection was 73%. Partial sternectomy was performed for primary sternal tumors when possible to obtain 5-cm margins. These patients had short hospitalization and good local control of the disease.[11]

SUMMARY

Chest wall resection requires wide local excision, negative margins, and adequate reconstruction. Outcomes are generally good to excellent with wide local excision and negative margins. Mortality is nearly 0% to 1% with mild morbidity. Multispecialty surgical teams may be required for more complex situations. Early diagnosis of chest wall sarcomas, confirmation by an experienced sarcoma pathologist, and multidisciplinary discussion before treatment initiation are all required for optimal and successful therapy.

REFERENCES

1. Walsh GL, Davis BM, Swisher SG, et al. A single-institutional, multidisciplinary approach to primary sarcomas involving the chest wall requiring full-thickness resections. J Thorac Cardiovasc Surg 2001;121:48–60.
2. Warzelhan J, Stoelben E, Imdahl A, et al. Results in surgery for primary and metastatic chest wall tumors. Eur J Cardiothorac Surg 2001;19:584–8.
3. Ryan MB, McMurtrey MJ, Roth JA. Current management of chest-wall tumors. Surg Clin North Am 1989; 69:1061–80.
4. Burt M, Fulton M, Wessner-Dunlap S, et al. Primary bony and cartilaginous sarcomas of chest wall: results of therapy. Ann Thorac Surg 1992;54: 226–32.
5. Sabanathan S, Shah R, Mearns AJ, et al. Chest wall resection and reconstruction. Br J Hosp Med 1997; 57:255–9.
6. Sabanathan S, Shah R, Mearns AJ. Surgical treatment of primary malignant chest wall tumours. Eur J Cardiothorac Surg 1997;11:1011–6.
7. Pairolero PC, Arnold PG. Chest wall tumors. Experience with 100 consecutive patients. J Thorac Cardiovasc Surg 1985;90:367–72.
8. Jeung MY, Gangi A, Gasser B, et al. Imaging of chest wall disorders. Radiographics 1999;19: 617–37.
9. Wyttenbach R, Vock P, Tschappeler H. Cross-sectional imaging with CT and/or MRI of pediatric chest tumors. Eur Radiol 1998;8:1040–6.
10. Hasse J. Reconstruction of chest wall defects. Thorac Cardiovasc Surg 1991;39(Suppl 3):241–7.
11. Soysal O, Walsh GL, Nesbitt JC, et al. Resection of sternal tumors: extent, reconstruction, and survival. Ann Thorac Surg 1995;60:1353–8.
12. McCormack P, Bains MS, Beattie EJ Jr, et al. New trends in skeletal reconstruction after resection of chest wall tumors. Ann Thorac Surg 1981;31:45–52.
13. Putnam JB Jr, Suell DM, Natarajan G, et al. Extended resection of pulmonary metastases: is the risk justified? Ann Thorac Surg 1993;55:1440–6.
14. Widhe B, Bauer HC. Scandinavian Sarcoma Group. Surgical treatment is decisive for outcome in chondrosarcoma of the chest wall: a population-based Scandinavian Sarcoma Group study of 106 patients. J Thorac Cardiovasc Surg 2009;137:610–4.

15. Mansour KA, Anderson TM, Hester TR. Sternal resection and reconstruction. Ann Thorac Surg 1993;55:838–42.

16. Grosfeld JL, Rescorla FJ, West KW, et al. Chest wall resection and reconstruction for malignant conditions in childhood. J Pediatr Surg 1988;23:667–73.

17. Shamberger RC, Grier HE. Chest wall tumors in infants and children. Semin Pediatr Surg 1994;3: 267–76.

18. Shamberger RC, Grier HE, Weinstein HJ, et al. Chest wall tumors in infancy and childhood. Cancer 1989;63:774–85.

19. Malangoni MA, Ofstein LC, Grosfeld JL, et al. Survival and pulmonary function following chest wall resection and reconstruction in children. J Pediatr Surg 1980;15:906–12.

20. Franken EA Jr, Smith JA, Smith WL. Tumors of the chest wall in infants and children. Pediatr Radiol 1977;6:13–8.

21. Andrassy RJ, Wiener ES, Raney RB, et al. Thoracic sarcomas in children. Ann Surg 1998;227:170–3.

22. Dang NC, Siegel SE, Phillips JD. Malignant chest wall tumors in children and young adults. J Pediatr Surg 1999;34:1773–8.

23. van den BH, van Rijn RR, Merks JH. Management of tumors of the chest wall in childhood: a review. J Pediatr Hematol Oncol 2008;30(3):214–21.

24. Hyans P, Moore JH Jr, Sinha L. Reconstruction of the chest wall with e-PTFE following major resection. Ann Plast Surg 1992;29:321–7.

25. Deschamps CM, Tirnaksiz BM, Darbandi R, et al. Early and long-term results of prosthetic chest wall reconstruction. J Thorac Cardiovasc Surg 1999; 117:588–92.

26. Martini N, Starzynski TE, Beattie EJ Jr. Problems in chest wall resection. Surg Clin North Am 1969;49: 313–22.

27. Eng J, Sabanathan S, Mearns AJ. Chest wall reconstruction after resection of primary malignant chest wall tumours. Eur J Cardiothorac Surg 1990;4:101–4.

28. Martini N, Huvos AG, Burt ME, et al. Predictors of survival in malignant tumors of the sternum. J Thorac Cardiovasc Surg 1996;111:96–105.

29. Seyfer AE, Graeber GM, Wind GG. Atlas of chest wall reconstruction. Rockville (MD): Aspen Publication; 1986. p. 1–260.

30. Graeber GM, Snyder RJ, Fleming AW, et al. Initial and long-term results in the management of primary chest wall neoplasms. Ann Thorac Surg 1982;34: 664–73.

31. Li G, Hansmann ML, Zwingers T, et al. Primary lymphomas of the lung: morphological, immunohistochemical and clinical features. Histopathology 1990;16:519–31.

32. Perry RR, Venzon D, Roth JA, et al. Survival after surgical resection for high-grade chest wall sarcomas. Ann Thorac Surg 1990;49:363–8.

33. Liptay MJ, Fry WA. Malignant bone tumors of the chest wall. Semin Thorac Cardiovasc Surg 1999; 11:278–84.

34. Eng J, Sabanathan S, Pradhan GN, et al. Primary bony chest wall tumours. J R Coll Surg Edinb 1990;35:44–7.

35. Patel SR, Burgess MA, Papadopoulos NE, et al. Extraskeletal myxoid chondrosarcoma. Long-term experience with chemotherapy. Am J Clin Oncol 1995;18:161–3.

36. Aoki J, Moser RP Jr, Kransdorf MJ. Chondrosarcoma of the sternum: CT features. J Comput Assist Tomogr 1989;13:806–10.

37. McAfee MK, Pairolero PC, Bergstralh EJ, et al. Chondrosarcoma of the chest wall: factors affecting survival. Ann Thorac Surg 1985;40:535–41.

38. Saenz NC, Hass DJ, Meyers P, et al. Pediatric chest wall Ewing's sarcoma. J Pediatr Surg 2000;35:550–5.

39. Seddon BM, Whelan JS. Emerging chemotherapeutic strategies and the role of treatment stratification in Ewing sarcoma. Paediatr Drugs 2008;10:93–105.

40. Shamberger RC, Laquaglia MP, Gebhardt MC, et al. Ewing sarcoma/primitive neuroectodermal tumor of the chest wall: impact of initial versus delayed resection on tumor margins, survival, and use of radiation therapy. Ann Surg 2003;238:563–7.

41. Jurgens H, Exner U, Gadner H, et al. Multidisciplinary treatment of primary Ewing's sarcoma of bone. A 6-year experience of a European Cooperative Trial. Cancer 1988;61:23–32.

42. Schuck A, Hofmann J, Rube C, et al. Radiotherapy in Ewing's sarcoma and PNET of the chest wall: results of the trials CESS 81, CESS 86 and EICESS 92. Int J Radiat Oncol Biol Phys 1998;42:1001–6.

43. Briccoli A, Rocca M, Salone M, et al. Local and systemic control of Ewing's bone sarcoma family tumors of the ribs. J Surg Oncol 2009;100:222–6.

44. Gordon MS, Hajdu SI, Bains MS, et al. Soft tissue sarcomas of the chest wall. Results of surgical resection. J Thorac Cardiovasc Surg 1991;101: 843–54.

45. Young MM, Kinsella TJ, Miser JS, et al. Treatment of sarcomas of the chest wall using intensive combined modality therapy. Int J Radiat Oncol Biol Phys 1989;16:49–57.

46. Goodlad JR, Mentzel T, Fletcher CD. Low grade fibromyxoid sarcoma: clinicopathological analysis of eleven new cases in support of a distinct entity. Histopathology 1995;26:229–37.

47. Kabiri EH, Al AS, El MA, et al. Desmoid tumors of the chest wall. Eur J Cardiothorac Surg 2001;19:580–3.

48. Hansmann A, Adolph C, Vogel T, et al. High-dose tamoxifen and sulindac as first-line treatment for desmoid tumors. Cancer 2004;100:612–20.

49. Raney RB Jr, Allen A, O'Neill J, et al. Malignant fibrous histiocytoma of soft tissue in childhood. Cancer 1986;57:2198–201.

50. Burt M, Karpeh M, Ukoha O, et al. Medical tumors of the chest wall. Solitary plasmacytoma and Ewing's sarcoma. J Thorac Cardiovasc Surg 1993; 105:89–96.

51. Tsukushi S, Nishida Y, Sugiura H, et al. Soft tissue sarcomas of the chest wall. J Thorac Oncol 2009;4:834–7.

52. Gokaslan ZL, York JE, Walsh GL, et al. Transthoracic vertebrectomy for metastatic spinal tumors. J Neurosurg 1998;89:599–609.

53. Walsh GL, Gokaslan ZL, McCutcheon IE, et al. Anterior approaches to the thoracic spine in patients with cancer: indications and results. Ann Thorac Surg 1997;64:1611–8.

54. Souba WW, McKenna RJ Jr, Meis J, et al. Radiation-induced sarcomas of the chest wall. Cancer 1986; 57:610–5.

55. Chapelier AR, Bacha EA, de Montpreville VT, et al. Radical resection of radiation-induced sarcoma of the chest wall: report of 15 cases. Ann Thorac Surg 1997;63:214–9.

56. Rustemeyer P, Micke O, Blasius S, et al. Radiation-induced malignant mesenchymoma of the chest wall following treatment for breast cancer. Br J Radiol 1997;70:424–6.

57. Schwarz RE, Burt M. Radiation-associated malignant tumors of the chest wall. Ann Surg Oncol 1996;3:387–92.

58. Neuhaus SJ, Pinnock N, Giblin V, et al. Treatment and outcome of radiation-induced soft-tissue sarcomas at a specialist institution. Eur J Surg Oncol 2009;35:654–9.

59. Gladdy RA, Qin LX, Moraco N, et al. Do radiation-associated soft tissue sarcomas have the same prognosis as sporadic soft tissue sarcomas? J Clin Oncol 2010;28:2064–9.

60. Korst RJ, Rosengart TK. Operative strategies for resection of pulmonary sarcomas extending into the left atrium. Ann Thorac Surg 1999;67: 1165–7.

61. Rickelt J, Hoekstra H, van CF, et al. Forequarter amputation for malignancy. Br J Surg 2009;96:792–8.

62. Wouters MW, van Geel AN, Nieuwenhuis L, et al. Outcome after surgical resections of recurrent chest wall sarcomas. J Clin Oncol 2008;26: 5113–8.

63. Incarbone M, Nava M, Lequaglie C, et al. Sternal resection for primary or secondary tumors. J Thorac Cardiovasc Surg 1997;114:93–9.

Muscle and Omental Flaps for Chest Wall Reconstruction

Mark T. Villa, MD, David W. Chang, MD*

KEYWORDS

- Chest wall • Reconstruction • Flaps

Reconstruction of the chest wall represents an important part of a patient's treatment after resection of a variety of thoracic tumors. Many different types of flaps, including both pedicled and free flaps, have been described for use in chest wall reconstruction. Pedicled muscle and myocutaneous options include the pectoralis major, latissimus dorsi, rectus abdominis, external oblique, and trapezius flaps. Omentum is another option that may be used either as a pedicled or free flap.

Reconstruction of chest wall defects can be, depending on the patient, a complicated undertaking and is best performed using a multidisciplinary approach. Preoperative planning is based on multiple factors that must be assessed and tailored to each patient to provide the best reconstruction possible. The assessment begins with the patient and includes prognosis, overall health, and both the desire and ability to undergo what can frequently be lengthy and difficult reconstructive procedures.

The type of reconstruction performed depends on several factors, including the size and exact location of the defect, the type of tissues resected, and the local conditions, such as previous radiotherapy or surgery, that may have compromised certain flap options. Superficial defects may be reconstructed with skin grafts. Resections involving deeper tissues may require flaps, as noted earlier. If appropriate local options have been compromised by prior surgery, if the defect is particularly large, or if there is extensive local injury from prior radiotherapy, free tissue transfer may be required.

Also, the surgeon may use tissue expansion to obtain larger flaps or temporize the flap site with subatmospheric pressure wound therapy.

MUSCLE AND MYOCUTANEOUS FLAPS
Pectoralis Major Flap

One of the most common options for reconstruction of chest wall defects is the pectoralis major muscle. This flap may be used as muscle only or may include a skin paddle. Pectoralis major muscle originates from the lateral aspect of the sternum and inserts into the intertubercular groove of the humerus. The muscle has 2 blood supplies: the dominant supply is the pectoral branch of the thoracoacromial trunk arising from the subclavian artery and the secondary supply consists of the second through sixth intercostal perforating vessels originating from the internal mammary artery. Venous drainage parallels the arterial supply. The dominant nerve supply to the muscle is the lateral pectoral nerve, with frequent smaller contributions from the medial pectoral nerve.

The flap may be raised based on either of its blood supplies. Basing the flap on the thoracoacromial vessels allows it to be raised as an island flap, which significantly increases its reach, particularly with division of the humeral insertion and clavicular origin. The reach may be further increased by burring down or even resecting a portion of the clavicle, which also helps to prevent any bulging that occurs when the muscle is transposed over the clavicle. Basing the flap

Financial disclosure: None.

Department of Plastic Surgery, University of Texas MD Anderson Cancer Center, 1515 Holcombe Boulevard, Unit 443, Houston, TX 77030, USA

* Corresponding author.

E-mail address: dchang@mdanderson.org

on the internal mammary perforating vessels allows for a turnover flap. The use of the turnover flap necessitates division of the humeral insertion, clavicular origin, and thoracoacromial vessels to allow for any mobility of the flap. The turnover flap represents a reasonable option that may be used for the reconstruction of midline defects, particularly in cases in which the thoracoacromial vessels are absent or damaged.

The pectoralis major flap has great utility for reconstruction of defects of the superior sternum and anterosuperior and anterolateral chest wall and neck. This flap may be used for external defects or passed between the superior ribs to occupy intrathoracic dead space that can result from partial or total lung resection (**Figs. 1–4**).

The flap may be raised as a muscle only or can include a skin island oriented vertically over the costochondral junction of the ribs or transversely at the inferior edge of the flap. Although the muscle flap is reliable, rates of skin paddle necrosis may be as high as 30%.[1–3] Additionally, loss of the anterior axillary fold can occur when the muscle is harvested in its entirety. Preservation of the lateral third of the muscle with the use of the medial two-thirds as a turnover flap can preserve the anterior axillary fold.[4]

Latissimus Dorsi Flap

Tansini[5] first described the use of the latissimus dorsi flap in 1906, and ever since it has become an important option for the reconstruction of chest wall defects. The latissimus dorsi muscle originates from the spinous processes of the 7th through 12th thoracic vertebrae and inserts into the intertubercular groove of the humerus. Its nerve supply is the thoracodorsal nerve and it has 2 blood supplies. The dominant blood supply is the thoracodorsal artery, which arises, in the large majority of patients, from the subscapular artery off the axillary artery. In a small percentage of individuals, the thoracodorsal artery arises from the axillary artery directly or from the lateral thoracic artery.[6] The secondary blood supply of the latissimus dorsi flap is the perforating vessels from the posterior intercostal vessels. Venous drainage parallels the arterial blood supply.

The average surface area of the latissimus dorsi flap has been shown to be 105 cm^2 in women and 195 cm^2 in men, which covers a defect of significant size.[7] The flap may be raised either as a muscle only or as a myocutaneous flap. Given the large surface area of the muscle, a significant amount of skin may be taken; however, one of the goals for this particular flap is that the donor site be closed primarily. Primary closure of the donor site is usually possible if the skin paddle is 10 cm or less; otherwise, skin grafting may be necessary. Tissue expansion has been described to increase the amount of skin available.[8,9]

As with the pectoralis major flap, the latissimus dorsi flap may be raised on its dominant or secondary blood supply. Also, as with the pectoralis flap, the choice of blood supply dictates the arc of rotation. Raising the flap on the thoracodorsal artery provides a significant amount of mobility, and the flap may be successfully used to cover almost any defect of the ipsilateral thorax, including the upper abdomen, head and neck, and upper extremity (**Figs. 5–7**). Certain strategies may be used, including disinserting the muscle from the humerus and aggressive dissection of the pedicle from its investing fascia, to increase the functional length of the flap.[10] The flap may also be passed between the ribs to occupy intrathoracic dead space.

Raising the latissimus dorsi flap on the intercostal perforators produces a turnover flap that can be used for the coverage of midline spinal defects, or the muscle may be dissected off the posterior chest wall, maintaining the perforating vessels, and advanced to cover more lateral chest wall defects if the thoracodorsal artery has been ligated. In the author's experience, an advancement of 6 to 8 cm is possible.

If there has been damage to the thoracodorsal pedicle, retrograde flow through the arterial supply of the serratus muscle into the thoracodorsal vessels may provide adequate blood supply to the flap to allow for division of the intercostal

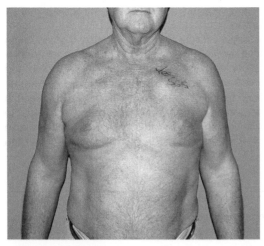

Fig. 1. Preoperative photo of a 68-year-old male with recurrent thymic carcinoma visible as a convexity to the left of the sternum.

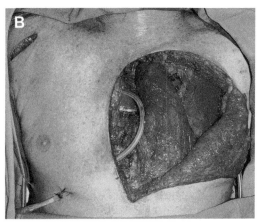

Fig. 2. (*A*) Intraoperative views of the patient whose resection included partial sternectomy, claviculectomy, and rib resection. (*B*) Demonstrates transposition of the turnover pectoralis flap to provide coverage of the great vessels.

perforators.[11] However, in patients with a history of radiotherapy, flap loss has been reported with use of a flap based on retrograde flow through the branch to the serratus.[12]

The skin paddle, if one is desired, may be oriented in several different ways on the back. The largest paddles are oriented with the long axis of the paddle parallel to the axis of the muscle. Other common orientations include a transverse orientation, with the idea that the scar may be hidden under a bra strap, or a crescentic skin paddle oriented within the relaxed skin tension lines of the back. Whatever the orientation, the scarring on the back can be prominent, and a contour abnormality may also be present after closure.

The latissimus dorsi myocutaneous flap has several disadvantages. Depending on the location of the chest wall defect, dissection of the flap may necessitate repositioning of the patient intraoperatively, which can lengthen operative time. An Achilles heel of this flap that has been reported postoperatively is a tendency toward seroma formation at the donor site, with one series reporting a 79% seroma rate as well as a donor site incision breakdown rate of 3%.[13,14] Surgeons can try to prevent seroma development by placing closed suction drains in the back and being conservative regarding their removal. Attempts to reduce seroma rates by using quilting sutures and fibrin sealants have been equivocally successful,[15] with quilting sutures appearing to be more effective than fibrin sealants.[16]

Perhaps the most important disadvantage of the latissimus dorsi myocutaneous flap is the functional deficits that occur in the ipsilateral arm. The

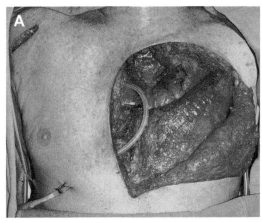

Fig. 3. Reconstruction of the defect using a left turnover pectoralis flap and a right islandized pectoralis major flap to provide adequate coverage of the great vessels and exposed lung.

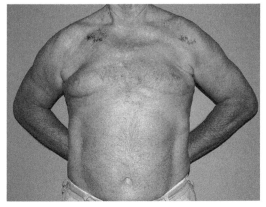

Fig. 4. Postoperative view of the patient, with stable coverage of vital structures.

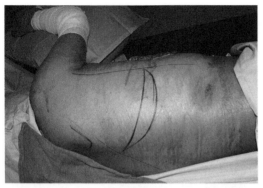

Fig. 5. Flap design for a right latissimus dorsi for chest wall reconstruction in a 58-year-old male with metastatic renal cell carcinoma.

most significant deficit is weakness of the arm, particularly on abduction between 90° and 180°. In the past, this deficit was thought to be minor; however, functional testing has demonstrated a reduction in arm strength, and this decrease in strength is more pronounced in women than in men.[17] More recent evidence suggests that although functional scores may be lower after harvest of the latissimus dorsi flap, this abnormality normalizes within 1 year postoperatively.[18] Some patients may demonstrate persistent back numbness and tightness after latissimus dorsi flap reconstruction.[19] For patients dependent on shoulder girdle strength for mobility, whether they are confined to a wheelchair or use a walker or crutches for ambulation, other alternatives that do not affect shoulder strength may be preferable to the use of the latissimus dorsi myocutaneous flap.

Rectus Abdominis Flaps

The rectus abdominis muscle originates from the pubis and inserts into the costal cartilages of the

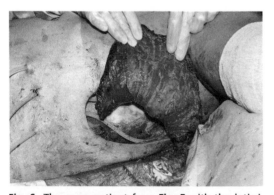

Fig. 6. The same patient from **Fig. 5** with the latissimus flap transposed anteriorly to cover the visible methyl methacrylate/Marlex mesh (Davol Inc, Cranston, RI, USA) construct used to reconstruct the chest wall defect.

fifth through seventh ribs and the xyphoid process. It is innervated segmentally by the thoracoabdominal nerves of T7-T12 vertebrae. Its arterial supply is from both the superior epigastric artery off the subclavian vessels and the inferior epigastric artery off the external iliac artery. The muscle may be isolated on either of these blood supplies.

Abdominal flaps based on the rectus abdominis muscle have become the mainstay of chest wall reconstruction for several reasons. These flaps provide a large amount of tissue; the skin paddles may be oriented transversely (transverse rectus abdominis myocutaneous [TRAM] flap), vertically (vertical rectus abdominis myocutaneous [VRAM] flap), or obliquely (oblique rectus abdominis myocutaneous flap); and the donor site can be closed primarily. The flap may also be pedicled on the superior epigastric vessels or transferred as a free flap based on the inferior epigastric vessels. This flexibility is of tremendous utility when reconstructing defects of the chest wall (**Figs. 8–10**).

The pedicled TRAM flap, based on the superior epigastric artery, was first described by Hartrampf and colleagues[20] in 1982. The transverse orientation of the skin paddle allows for a large amount of tissue to be harvested from a site that can be closed primarily, while producing a relatively inconspicuous scar. The blood supply to the skin and subcutaneous tissues comes from perforators off the epigastric system. The superior and inferior epigastric vessels connect through a choke zone periumbilically. The vertical orientation of the VRAM flap skin paddle maximizes the number of perforating vessels supplying the skin, providing a more robust blood supply to the skin paddle than the TRAM flap. Problems can arise for chest wall reconstruction if the internal mammary vessels have been resected; however, the flap may be based on the contributions of the eighth intercostal vessel to the epigastric system. This arrangement, however, provides decreased vascularity to the flap.[21]

The initial description of the rectus abdominis flap divided the abdominal tissues into zones 1 to 4 based on the blood supply. Zone 1 lay immediately over the rectus muscle being harvested, zone 2 lay adjacent to zone 1 on the contralateral side of the abdomen, zone 3 was lateral to zone 1, and zone 4 was lateral to zone 2. Subsequent investigation into the blood supply of the abdomen has led to modifications of these classifications of the abdominal zones. The present thinking is that zone 1 is as described earlier, zone 2 is lateral to zone 1, zone 3 is immediately adjacent to zone 1 on the contralateral side of the abdomen, and zone 4 is lateral to zone 3.[22]

Many methods of augmenting the blood supply to the TRAM skin paddle have been described.

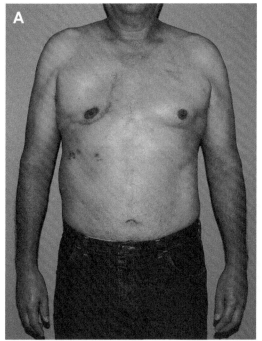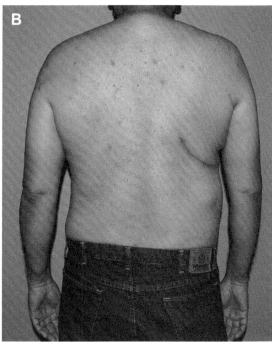

Fig. 7. Anterior (*A*) and posterior (*B*) postoperative views showing well-healed incisions and stable coverage.

These include harvesting both rectus abdominis muscles and the so-called supercharging a pedicled TRAM flap by performing microvascular anastomosis of the deep or superficial inferior epigastric vessels to recipient vessels in the chest.

Donor site morbidity for abdominal flaps can take the form of weakness,[23] abdominal bulges (3.8%), or hernias (2.6%).[24] The deep inferior epigastric perforator (DIEP) flap and the superficial inferior epigastric (SIEA) flap represent the 2 means by which the muscle and fascia of the abdominal wall may be spared. Comparisons of donor site morbidity for muscle-sparing TRAM and DIEP flaps have demonstrated no functional difference in abdominal morbidity.[25] The SIEA flap has been shown to cause less abdominal morbidity than either the muscle-sparing TRAM or the DIEP flap.[26]

External Oblique Flap

The external oblique muscle originates from the lower 8 ribs and inserts into the inguinal ligament and the iliac crest. Its blood supply comes from the lateral cutaneous branches of the 8 inferoposterior intercostal arteries. These arteries enter the muscle posteriorly and provide a segmental blood supply to the muscle. In addition, these vessels send perforating branches to the overlying skin. Thus, the external oblique flap may be used as

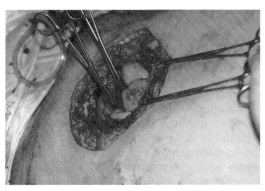

Fig. 8. Full-thickness anterior chest wall defect.

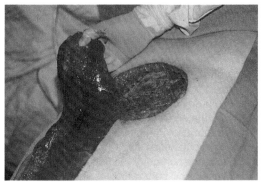

Fig. 9. Chest wall reconstructed with Marlex mesh and pedicled TRAM flap.

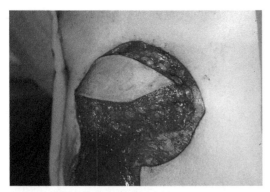

Fig. 10. A pedicled TRAM flap.

a myofascial or myocutaneous flap that can be used to cover defects located in the lower anterior chest up to the level of the third intercostal space.[27]

In the past, the description of the dissection of this flap included the anterior rectus sheath.[28] Although this fascia may serve a purpose in the reconstruction of the chest wall, it can necessitate the use of prosthetic or bioprosthetic mesh for donor site closure. It has since been demonstrated that the flap may be safely raised without the anterior rectus sheath, which helps to limit the donor site morbidity of this flap and obviates the need for a mesh.[29] During the dissection, the surgeon establishes the plane between the external and internal obliques medially at the linea semilunaris. The surgeon then carries the dissection laterally until the neurovascular bundles from the intercostal vessels are encountered.

Trapezius Flap

The trapezius is a broad diamond-shaped muscle located on the posterior thorax. It has multiple origins including the external occipital protuberance, the nuchal ligament, the medial superior nuchal line, and the C7-T12 spinous processes. The trapezius also has several insertions: the lateral third of the clavicle, the acromion process, and the scapular spine. Its arterial supply is predominantly the transverse cervical artery arising from the thyrocervical trunk that, in turn, arises off the subclavian artery. Its neural supply is via the 11th cranial nerve, the spinal accessory. It is useful for coverage of defects in the upper midback, the neck, and the shoulders.

The trapezius flap may be raised as a muscular or musculocutaneous flap. The blood supply to the cutaneous portion of the flap consists of musculocutaneous perforators. The cutaneous portion of the flap may extend well below the level of the muscle itself, provided that one-third of the skin paddle lies over the muscle.[30] If raised as a musculocutaneous flap, a skin paddle of less than 10 cm enables primary closure of the donor site.

Morbidity of the flap is low, provided that the surgeon preserves the superior 4 cm of the muscle, the spinal accessory nerve, and the insertion at the acromion.

Free Tissue Transfer

Although multiple local options exist for chest wall reconstruction, as noted previously, the availability of these options may be limited by several local factors, including trauma and prior radiotherapy or surgery, particularly in patients with recurrent disease.

Although local options represent the first choice for most patients, for certain patients, free flap reconstruction of the chest wall may be required.[31] Many of the flaps described earlier may be used for free tissue transfer, including the latissimus dorsi, rectus abdominis, and omental flaps. Free tissue transfer also allows for the use of common lower extremity flaps, including the anterolateral thigh flap and the vastus lateralis flap.

Multiple recipient vessels are available, including the internal mammary vessels, the thoracodorsal and lateral thoracic vessels, and the branches of the thoracoacromial and thyrocervical trunks.

As noted, most patients do not require a free tissue transfer. Also, some patients requiring chest wall reconstruction may be poor candidates for a free flap owing either to a poor prognosis or medical comorbidities. However, in appropriately chosen patients, microsurgery expands the repertoire of flaps available for reconstruction of the chest wall.

OMENTAL FLAPS

The greater omentum consists of a large fold of peritoneum that is associated with the transverse colon and the greater curvature of the stomach. In addition to peritoneum, it contains variable amounts of fat and lymphoid tissue. An extensive vascular network, with contributions from the right and left gastroepiploic arteries as well as the short gastric vessels, supplies the blood to the omentum.

The large number of vessels supplying the omentum provides tremendous flexibility with regard to flap design. For low midline defects, all of the vascular supplies may be left intact. However, owing to its extensive vascular arcade, the omentum may be isolated on the right or left gastroepiploic vessels after division of both its

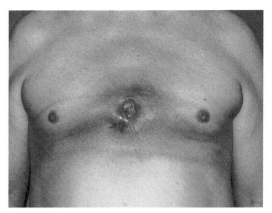

Fig. 11. Preoperative view showing a large chondrosarcoma of the sternal body in a 47-year-old male.

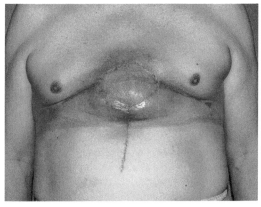

Fig. 13. The omental flap with a well-healed skin graft at approximately 4 months postoperation.

attachments to the transverse colon and division of the short gastric vessels.[32] This procedure provides a large pedicled flap that may be readily used with a skin graft for reconstruction of the chest wall in almost any location (**Figs. 11–13**).

Several disadvantages exist with the use of the omental flap. Harvest requires a laparotomy, although laparoscopic harvest has been described.[33] In addition, passage of the omentum

into the chest wall defect via a subcutaneous tunnel can result in the development of a hernia, which may be ameliorated by using a transdiaphragmatic passage of the omentum.[34] The omentum can also be flimsy, small, or absent if previous abdominal surgeries have been performed, which can complicate or even prohibit its use for reconstruction of the chest wall.

SUMMARY

Multiple options, both local and distant, exist for the reconstruction of chest wall defects. The type of reconstruction depends on multiple factors including patient health and motivation and previous treatments, both medical and surgical. These reconstructions are most effectively managed with a multidisciplinary approach involving plastic and cardiothoracic surgeries. As noted earlier, the pectoralis major, latissimus dorsi, rectus abdominis, trapezius, and external oblique muscles and the omentum are all local options that can play an important role in the reconstruction of the chest wall. They may be used individually or in combination to provide adequate tissue bulk and surface area for these important, and often difficult, reconstructions.

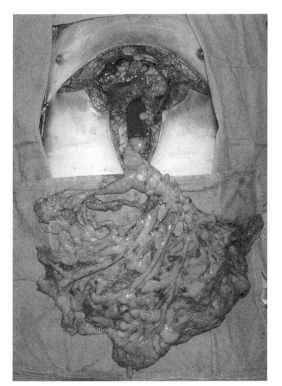

Fig. 12. Intraoperative view showing the defect of the lower sternum and surrounding costal cartilages with the omental flap after harvest.

REFERENCES

1. Mehta S, Sarkar S, Kavarana N, et al. Complications of the pectoralis major myocutaneous flap in the oral cavity: a prospective evaluation of 220 cases. Plast Reconstr Surg 1996;98:31–7.
2. Kroll S, Reece G, Miller M, et al. Comparison of the rectus abdominis free flap with the pectoralis major myocutaneous flap for reconstruction in the head and neck. Am J Surg 1992;164:615–8.
3. Castelli M, Pecorari G, Succo G, et al. Pectoralis major myocutaneous flaps: analysis of complications in

difficult patients. Eur Arch Otorhinolaryngol 2001; 258:542–5.

4. Nahai F, Morales L, Bone D, et al. Pectoralis major muscle turnover flaps or closure of the infected sternotomy wound with preservation of form and function. Plast Reconstr Surg 1982;70:471–4.

5. Tansini I. Sopra il mio nuovo proceso di amputazione della mamella. Gazz Med Ital Torino 1906;57:141 [in Italian].

6. Roswell A, Eisenberg N, Davies D, et al. The anatomy of the thoracodorsal artery within the latissimus dorsi muscle. Br J Plast Surg 1986;39:206–9.

7. Serafin D. The latissimus dorsi muscle – musculocutaneous flap. In: Serafin D, editor. Atlas of microsurgical composite tissue transplantation. Philadelphia: WB Saunders; 1996. p. 208.

8. Slavin S. Improving the latissimus dorsi myocutaneous flap with tissue expansion. Plast Reconstr Surg 1994;98:811–24.

9. Motamed S, Kalantar-Hormozi A, Marzban S. Expanded occipito-cervico-pectoral flap for reconstruction of burned cervical contracture. Burns 2003;29:842–4.

10. Mathes S. Latissimus dorsi. In: Mathes SJ, Nahai F, editors. Principles of reconstructive surgery. St Louis (MO): Quality Medical Publishing; 1998. p. 478–94.

11. Fisher J, Bostwick J, Powell R. Latissimus dorsi blood supply after thoracodorsal blood vessel division: the serratus collateral. Plast Reconstr Surg 1983;72:502–11.

12. Salmon R, Razaboni R, Soussaline M. The use of the latissimus dorsi musculocutaneous flap following recurrence of cancer in irradiated breasts. Br J Surg 1988;41:41–4.

13. Delay E, Gounot N, Bouillot A, et al. Autologous latissimus dorsi breast reconstruction: a 3-year clinical experience with 100 patients. Plast Reconstr Surg 1998;102:1461–78.

14. Menke H, Erkens M, Olbrisch R. Evolving concepts in breast reconstruction with latissimus dorsi flaps: results and follow up of 121 consecutive patients. Ann Plast Surg 2001;47:107–14.

15. Titley O, Spyrou G, Fatah M. Preventing seroma in the latissimus dorsi flap donor site. Br J Plast Surg 1997;50:106–8.

16. Akhtar S, Syrou G, Fourie L. Our early experience in the use of tissue glue to reduce the incidence of seroma formation from the latissimus dorsi donor site. Plast Reconstr Surg 2005;116(1):347–8.

17. Fraulin F, Louie G, Sorrilla L, et al. Functional evaluation of the shoulder following latissimus dorsi muscle transfer. Ann Plast Surg 1995;35: 349–55.

18. Glassey N, Perks G, McCulley S. A prospective assessment of shoulder morbidity and recovery time scales following latissimus dorsi breast reconstruction. Plast Reconstr Surg 2008;122: 1334–40.

19. Adams W, Lipschitz A, Ansari M, et al. Funtional donor site morbidity following latissimus dorsi muscle flap transfer. Ann Plast Surg 1995;53:349–55.

20. Hartrampf C, Scheflan M, Balck P, et al. Breast reconstruction with a transverse abdominal island flap. Plast Reconstr Surg 1982;69(2):216–24.

21. Paletta C, Vogler G, Freedman B. Viability of the rectus abdominis muscle following internal mammary artery ligation. Plast Reconstr Surg 1993;92:234–7.

22. Holm C, Mayr M, Hofter E, et al. Perfusion zones of the DIEP flap revisited: a clinical study. Plast Reconstr Surg 2006;117(1):37–43.

23. Blondeel P, Vanderstraeten G, Monstrey S, et al. The donor site morbidity of free DIEP flaps and free TRAM flaps for breast reconstruction. Br J Plast Surg 1997;50:322–30.

24. Kroll S, Schusterman M, Reece G, et al. Abdominal wall strength, bulging, and hernia after TRAM flap breast reconstruction. Plast Reconstr Surg 1995; 96:616–9.

25. Bajaj A, Chevray P, Chang D. Comparison of donor-site complications and functional outcomes in free muscle-sparing TRAM flap and DIEP flap breast reconstruction. Plast Reconstr Surg 2006;117(3): 737–46.

26. Wu L, Bajaj A, Chang D, et al. Comparison of donor-site morbidity of SIEA, DIEP, and muscle-sparing TRAM flaps for breast reconstruction. Plast Reconstr Surg 2008;122(3):702–9.

27. Bogossian N, Chaglassian T, Rosenberg P, et al. External oblique myocutaneous flap coverage of large chest wall defects following resection of breast tumors. Plast Reconstr Surg 1996;97:97–103.

28. Marshall D, Anstee E, Stapleton M. Post-mastectomy breast reconstruction using a direct flap from an abdominal lipectomy. Br J Plast Surg 1981;34:280–5.

29. Moschella F, Cordova A. A new extended external oblique musculocutaneous flap for reconstruction of large chest wall defects. Plast Reconstr Surg 1999;103:1378–85.

30. Cormack G, Lamberty G. Trunk. In: The arterial anatomy of skin flaps. New York: Churchill Livingstone; 1994. p. 132–48.

31. Hidalgo D, Saldana E, Rusch V. Free flap chest wall reconstruction for recurrent breast cancer and radiation ulcers. Ann Plast Surg 1993;30:375–80.

32. Das S. The size of the human omentum and methods of lengthening it for transposition. Br J Plast Surg 1976;29:144–70.

33. Acarturk T, Swatz W, Luketich J, et al. Laparoscopically harvested omental flap for chest wall and intrathoracic reconstruction. Ann Plast Surg 2004;53:210–6.

34. Weinzweig N, Yetman R. Transposition of the greater omentum for recalcitrant median sternotomy wound infections. Ann Plast Surg 1995;34:471–7.

Prosthetic Reconstruction of the Chest Wall

Pascal A. Thomas, MD[a],*, Laurent Brouchet, MD, PhD[b]

KEYWORDS

- Chest wall reconstruction • Osteosynthesis
- Methyl methacrylate prosthesis

The oncologic concept of en bloc resection ensuring healthy margins does not have any compromise (Video 1; www.thoracic.theclinics.com). However, large full-thickness chest wall defects produce skeletal instability that impacts on the respiratory mechanics, the consequences of which should considered along with the individual patient's baseline pulmonary status or the possible combined lung resection. The ensuing "paradoxical breathing" is all the more important because the resection is wide, typically with a minimum of three ribs involved, and its location is anterior, especially if the sternum is concerned. Besides the restoration of the skeletal rigidity, chest wall reconstruction has five additional objectives: (1) to avoid that the chest wall defect entails a lung hernia (Video 2; www.thoracic.theclinics.com), (2) to counteract substantial shrinking of the operated side of the thorax, leading to a thoracoplasty-like effect, (3) to prevent impaction of the scapula in case of posterior chest wall resections, especially when the resection is extended down to 5th and 6th ribs, (4) to protect the underlying mediastinal organs against external impact, especially after sternal resection, and (5) to maintain a good cosmetic chest shape.

Because no precise guidelines exist in the literature on the size and location of defects that absolutely necessitate restoration of the continuity of the bony framework, none exist either regarding the ideal materials to be used. Moreover, composite reconstructions mixing several prosthetic materials, covered with those autologous muscular, musculocutaneous, or omental flaps needed to manage simultaneously the soft tissues resection, are mostly required for large defect reconstructions. However, the functional, mechanical, and protective benefits of rigid prosthetic chest wall reconstruction should be balanced against the risks of infection in each individual patient, depending on the underlying condition and its previous treatments (eg, chemotherapy, radiotherapy) and the presence of predisposing comorbidities.

The reconstruction now occurs immediately after the resection, which has contributed toward improving recovery and outcome. Thus, planning of the ablative and reconstructive stages of the operation is of paramount importance to tailor the various reconstructive options to the extent of resection. This article focuses only on the currently available options for the chest wall reconstruction using prosthetic materials.

AVAILABLE MATERIALS AND TECHNIQUES

The use of metal prostheses was first reported by a French surgeon Gangolphe[1] in 1909. In the 1940s, better-tolerated and easier-to-use materials emerged, such as tantalum plates,[2] but the modern era of chest wall reconstruction arose with the advent of plastic components.[3] In 1960, Graham and colleagues[4] provided a comprehensive historical perspective of these early steps.

[a] Department of Thoracic Surgery, University Hospitals of Marseille, University of the Mediterranean, Marseille, France
[b] Department of Thoracic Surgery, Rangueil-Larrey University Hospital, Toulouse, France
* Corresponding author. Department of Thoracic Surgery, North University Hospital, Chemin des Bourrely, 13326 Marseille Cedex 20, France.
E-mail address: pathomas@ap-hm.fr

Thorac Surg Clin 20 (2010) 551–558
doi:10.1016/j.thorsurg.2010.06.006
1547-4127/10/$ – see front matter © 2010 Elsevier Inc. All rights reserved.

Half a century later, a multitude of materials exists, including synthetic meshes, bone substitutes, osteosynthesis systems, and dedicated plastic or metallic prostheses. Although these all have specific advantages and disadvantages, all seem to work satisfactorily, and most of them may be combined for composite reconstructions of challenging situations. They more or less all comply with the characteristics of the ideal prosthetic material, as determined by Le Roux and Shama[5]: (1) rigidity to abolish paradoxical movement, (2) inertness to allow in-growth of fibrous tissue and decrease the likelihood of infection, (3) malleability so that it can be fashioned to the appropriate shape at the time of operation, and (4) radiolucency to create an anatomic reference to identify possible local relapse of the primary disease at radiographic follow-up. Therefore, the choice of a prosthetic material is puzzling and, for the most part, has been based mainly on the surgeon's preference and some cost-effective concerns.

Meshes and Patches

Meshes and patches are easily manipulated and handled. They are usually doubled over and sutured to adjacent ribs and fascia to cover the immediate surface of the chest wall defect. When appropriate, the sutures penetrate the rib with a large needle or a special punch rather than the muscle only, which can get torn. These materials can be stretched uniformly in all directions, thereby allowing uniform distribution of tension at the skeletal defect edges (**Fig. 1**). They are simple to suture and mold into the wound. Interstices of knitted meshes render them permeable to body fluids and prevent the occurrence of seroma.

However, patches provide a barrier that prevents fluid and air from moving between the pleural and subcutaneous space. They usually have long-lasting tolerability without notable foreign-body reactions. They also propose a scaffold for the in-growth of regenerative connective tissue colonizing their outer and inner surfaces, and this remodeling process also provides appropriate stability of the chest wall. However, even if these patches offer reasonable tension resistance, the strength is not always sufficient to protect underlying endothoracic organs from an external impact in case of an anterior location, even when stretched as a drum. They also cannot be shaped according to the roundness of the lateral chest wall after large resections.

Most patches are nonabsorbable synthetic woven meshes: polypropylene (Marlex, Davol & Bard, Cranston, RI, USA and Prolene, Ethicon, Inc, Somerville, NJ, USA), polyesther (Mersilene, Ethicon, Inc, Somerville, NJ, USA), and polytetrafluoroethylene soft tissue patches (Gore-Tex & Gore-Dualmesh, W.L. Gore & Associates, Inc, Flagstaff, AZ, USA), or, more recently, knitted meshes (Gore-Tex, W.L. Gore & Associates, Inc, Flagstaff, AZ, USA). The Vicryl (polyglactin-910) mesh (Ethicon, Inc, Somerville, NJ, USA) is an inert, nonantigenic, biocompatible, and slowly absorbing material, the last being the main rationale for its use in patients at risk of suppuration. Synthetic meshes as a whole are simple to use and usually well tolerated when completely covered by viable tissue, at a reasonable cost.

Biologic meshes, as those based on bovine pericardium (Tutomesh, Tutogen Medical, Inc, Alachua, FL, USA), have the same tensile strength and elasticity as those of synthetic meshes and proper physiologic properties, which make them more resistant to infection and contamination. They consist of acellular organic collagen-based matrices, and seem especially useful in contaminated fields because they allow for native tissue regrowth and revascularization, stimulating regeneration as opposed to scarring, with minimal inflammatory response and less inclination toward rejection. Their main limitation is their cost.

Methyl Methacrylate

Methyl methacrylate (Simplex P, Stryker Howmedica Osteonics, Mahwah, NJ, USA) is usually sandwiched between two layers of mesh to strengthen the rigidity of the reconstruction. This material has gained increasing popularity since the early 1980s, because it allows a customized bridging of virtually every skeletal chest wall defect.[6] The prosthesis is typically prepared and shaped back-table (**Fig. 2**).

Lardinois and colleagues[7] brought sound modifications to the conventional technique. After resection of the chest wall, the first and inner

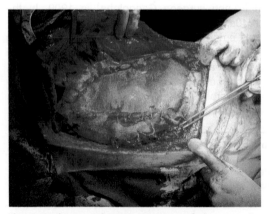

Fig. 1. Prolene mesh reconstruction of the posterior chest wall. The scapula is retracted by a hook.

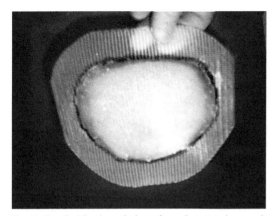

Fig. 2. Sandwiched methyl methacrylate Marlex mesh prosthesis. The size of the prosthesis is tailored to the one of the chest wall defect to be bridged.

mesh is sutured under tension to bridge the defect. The viscosity of methyl methacrylate is also lowered by mixing 40 g of polymeric powder with 30 mL instead of 20 mL liquid monomer, leading to a longer time required for hardening. The methyl methacrylate is then applied in situ on the fixed mesh and modeled to the resection margins of the chest wall (**Fig. 3**). The second and external mesh is then integrated in the methyl methacrylate, still in its viscous phase, and tightly anchored to the chest wall. The prosthesis is finally continuously cooled by irrigation with water during hardening to prevent heat injury to adjacent structures. During this process, the underlying lung is kept ventilated with positive end-expiratory pressure and normal tidal volumes to simulate the natural shape of the chest wall to be replaced. These modifications allow a better configuration of the prosthesis, leading to better functional and cosmetic results and fewer substitute dislocations from optimal anchorage of the prosthesis in the surrounding tissue.

Whatever the application technique, methyl methacrylate results in very rigid chest wall substitutes. This mechanical quality may also become a problem when altering the physiologic movements of the rib cage in large defect reconstructions. Methyl methacrylate also generates the formation of seroma in the surrounding soft tissues, which make a favorable medium for infection.

Another technique is to shape neo-ribs, as thoroughly described by Dahan and colleagues.[8] For this procedure requires silicone molds for reproducing the typical outlines of a rib. After chest wall resection, the costal margins are made anfractuous with the use of rodent pliers. Kirschner's wires are then inserted into the spongiest aspect of the cut ribs and curved at their free extremities. The silicone molds are threaded on ribs and wires, and tied tight with ligatures at both extremities. Methyl methacrylate, still in its viscous phase, is injected in the mold to fill it totally. As soon as the hardening is gained, the mold is split and removed. Finally, possible harshness at the neo-ribs surface is polished (**Fig. 4**).

Similar technique may be used for partial sternal replacement. This technique provides excellent stability but also offers a suitable support to receive a regional (**Fig. 5**) or omental flap while allowing some tissue in-growth and better fluid drainage from the chest wall soft tissues into the pleural space than does a nonporous large plate of methyl methacrylate. It also allows easy radiographic follow-up (**Fig. 6**).

Osteosynthesis Systems

Osteosynthesis systems are rarely used alone in the setting of chest wall reconstruction after wide resections. However, they offer an ingenious and ergonomic solution to complex problems that

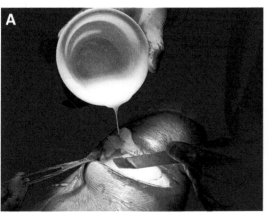

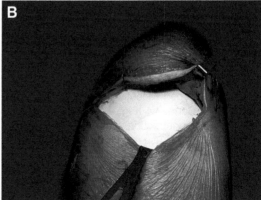

Fig. 3. Methyl methacrylate chest wall reconstruction. (*A*) Methyl methacrylate is applied in situ on a fixed mesh and (*B*) modeled to the resection margins of the chest wall.

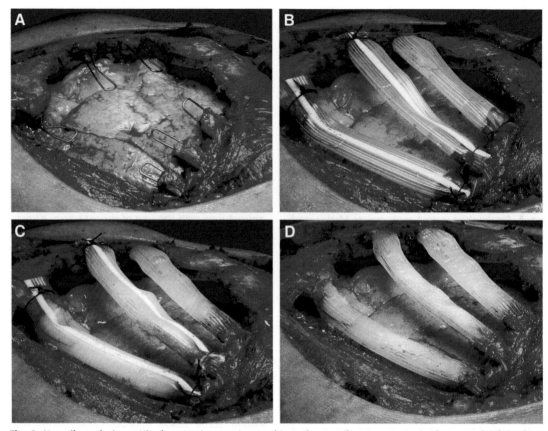

Fig. 4. Neo-ribs technique. Kirschner's wires are inserted into the cut ribs, to serve as the framework of the foreseen reconstruction (*A*). The silicone molds are threaded on ribs and wires, and tight with ligatures at both extremities (*B*). Methyl methacrylate, still in its viscous phase, is injected in the mold to fill it totally (*C*). The molds are finally split and removed (*D*).

necessitate multistage rib bridging or anterior chest wall stabilization. Numerous materials and systems exist. One of the oldest dedicated ones in this indication is the Borrelly steel staple-splints system (Medicalex, Bagneux, France).[9] This pioneer system includes a set of rib staples, splints of different length, straight and angular connectors allowing all kind of assemblies to be tailored to the needs of a given operation, and a dedicated ancillary material with crimping pliers for the staplers and the sliding connectors, and camber pliers for the splints. A very conceptually similar system, with a titanium implantable material, was developed recently (Stratos, MedXpert, Heitersheim, Germany) (**Fig. 7**) and reported for chest wall reconstruction, but with a greater cost-in-use.[10] The use of titanium has several advantages. It is highly corrosion-resistant and has the highest strength/weight ratio of any metal, and is biologically well tolerated and can integrate with bone. Its nonferromagnetic properties allow implanted patients to be examined with MRI. Other osteosynthesis systems with plates and

screws (**Fig. 8**), initially developed for a more ubiquitous use than the two previous ones, now include titanium materials (Titanium Sternal Fixation System, Synthes, Solothurn, Switzerland), and their use has been widely reported for these indications.[11–13]

To summarize, osteosynthesis systems provides a good basement reconstructive frame for large chest wall defects. They are thus commonly used with meshes or patches, and regional or omental flaps. Reestablishing the individual rib continuity allows more physiologic rib movements than larger fixed methyl methacrylate prosthesis. However, they may generate all of the complications seen with those materials in other sites, such as rupture, displacement, and infection.

Dedicated Sternal Prostheses

The Ley prosthesis is a 0.5-mm thick titanium alloy plate shaped as a stepladder. It is flexible and adapts to the sternal contour. This device has

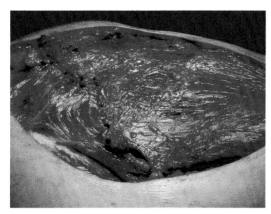

Fig. 5. Neo-ribs prosthesis coverage. The neo-ribs prosthesis is covered by a pectoralis major muscle transposition.

been initially designed for stabilization of the sternum after postoperative mediastinitis and in aseptic chronic sternal dehiscence. A recent report showed it was used successfully in three patients after resection of sternal chondrosarcoma.[14]

Watanabe and colleagues[15] reported on the use of a sternal ceramic prosthesis composed of hydroxyapatite and tricalcium phosphate (Ceratite, NGK Spark Plug Co, Aichi, Japan). It consists of a customized prosthetic bone that can be tailored to the anterior chest wall defect by cutting slots and holes in the Ceratite prosthesis for use as fasteners. This concept is original, and the component material has several advantages, such as the ability to provide the appropriate template for bone formation, strength, and biocompatibility. Its main disadvantage is its cost.

RESULTS

A review of the literature on prosthetic chest wall reconstruction is hampered by several limitations, the strongest of which is the absence of

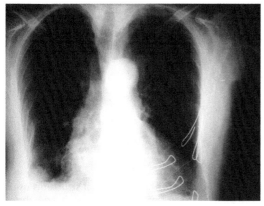

Fig. 6. Neo-ribs technique. Postoperative chest radiograph.

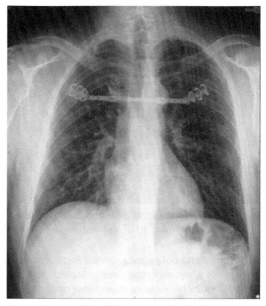

Fig. 7. Chest wall stabilization with a bridging osteosynthesis Stratos system after partial sternectomy. Postoperative chest radiograph.

prospective trials comparing the different techniques and materials because of the low surgical volume, even in specialized centers. Furthermore, most single-institution experiences encompass multiple decades, and therefore do not optimally show the continuous refinements in patient selection, surgical technique, reconstructive materials, and postoperative care. Furthermore, some outcomes, such as patient quality of life and cosmetic considerations, have seldom been measured scientifically but are often postulated.

The clinical impact of prosthetic reconstruction after chest wall resection is primarily extrapolated from the treatment of traumatic flail chest, which suggests that patients with large flail segments benefit from chest wall stabilization, which in turn decreases pulmonary complications and length of ventilatory support.[16]

Respiratory complications continue to be the main source of morbidity after chest wall resection, and include atelectasis, pneumonia, and acute respiratory distress syndrome that have been reported to be as high as 20% to 25%.[17,18] These complications remain the principal cause of death after chest wall resection, accounting for approximately 5% of deaths.[19–21] A contemporary experience from the Memorial Sloan-Kettering Cancer Center[19] showed that the incidence of respiratory complications could be halved, but whether careful selection for use of a rigid prosthesis minimized the incidence of these postoperative respiratory complications was unclear.

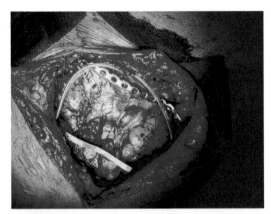

Fig. 8. Chest wall stabilization with a titanium osteo-synthesis system after partial sternectomy.

Lardinois and colleagues[7] presented convincing arguments when reporting their prospective experience with 26 patients who underwent chest wall resection and reconstruction with Marlex mesh methyl methacrylate sandwiches, showing no mortality and no significant difference in preoperative and postoperative forced expiratory volume at 1 second, even among patients undergoing concomitant lung resections. Moreover, in a contemporaneous series of 92 consecutive patients who had undergone reconstruction of the thoracic wall, of whom two-thirds received a nonrigid Prolene mesh for stabilization, most long-term survivors experienced sensation disorders and motion-dependent pain, which contributed significantly to hypoxemia.[20]

Although rigid prostheses provide excellent chest wall stability and a possibly lowered risk of respiratory complications, they are associated with a greater number of wound complications, especially methyl methacrylate-based ones, than those associated with nonrigid prostheses.[21] Wound complications, such as hematoma, seroma, infection, and delayed wound healing, are reported to occur in 10% to 20% of patients at 90 days, and require removal of the material in approximately 5%.[19] However, whether these wound complications primarily relate to the kind of prosthesis or to confounders, such as the size

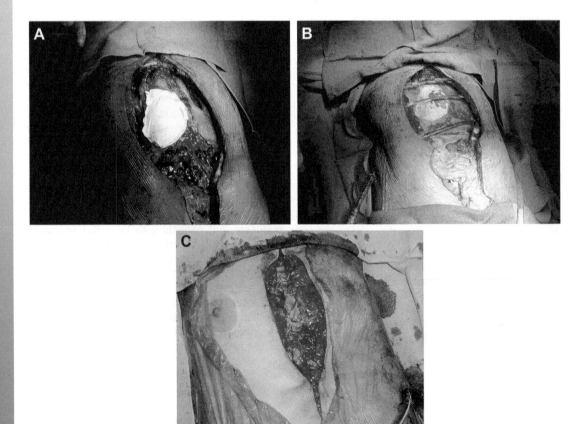

Fig. 9. Total sternectomy for a radiation-induced bone sarcoma. Protection of the mediastinal structures using a polytetrafluoroethylene patch. (A) Chest wall stabilization using the association Prolene mesh and three-stage osteosynthesis Borrelly system (B). Soft tissue reconstruction with an omental flap sustained by preceding synthetic mesh (C).

of the chest wall defects or the type of soft tissue transposition for coverage, is impossible to determine within the context of these retrospective studies.

DISCUSSION

Posterior and apical chest wall defects generally do not require prosthetic reconstruction for functional reasons because of the natural parietal suspension provided by the sternum, scapula, clavicula, and attached wide muscles of the thorax. However, defects that extend down to 5th and 6th ribs may cause the impaction of the tip of the scapula, which is a source of discomfort. In those patients, bridging the defect through suturing a synthetic mesh under tension is adequate. Small lateral or anterior defects of the rib cage that are likely to produce lung herniation may be reconstructed accordingly. Conversely, large lateral resections and most anterior defects that both engender paradoxical chest wall motion require rigid reconstruction.

For laterally located defects, the cheapest and most used option is methyl methacrylate sandwiched between two layers of mesh. For very large defects, composite reconstructions with meshes and cross-hatching strips of methyl methacrylate or the neo-ribs technique, rather than creating an entirely solid plate, seem preferable to prevent wound complications. Alternative composite options using osteosynthesis systems undoubtedly enable faster progress but are more expensive.

Anterior defects involving the sternum totally or subtotally are more demanding to reconstruct because of the strong mechanical constraints in this area and the vulnerability of the underlying mediastinal structures to external impact. Dedicated prostheses are surely elegant but expensive and currently poorly available materials. Furthermore, they do not apply to wide parietal resections extending laterally to the sternum. This area is perhaps the best place for a three-layer reconstruction (**Fig. 9**), with a first internal polytetrafluoroethylene patch that minimizes tissue attachment with the heart and great vessels along its inner surface, then a rigid stabilization either with bridging methyl methacrylate or osteosynthesis, and finally associated with a synthetic knitted mesh to encourage host tissue in-growth. This type of major procedure may be performed with very satisfactory cosmetic results (**Fig. 10**).

Contaminated wounds have few areas for one-stage chest wall resection and prosthetic reconstruction, typically requiring autologous tissue transpositions only. However, when surgeons believe that patients cannot be extubated in a reasonable time without additional support, an absorbable or biologic mesh may contribute to early stabilization.

SUMMARY

The choice of techniques and materials for chest wall reconstruction depends on the size and position of the defect, the surgeon's proper experience, and some economical considerations. Meanwhile, the availability of multiple, possibly combined, more adapted, and better-tolerated prostheses have pushed past the limits of resection to those involving soft tissue coverage, an issue that is addressed in another article.

APPENDIX: SUPPLEMENTARY DATA

Supplementary data associated with this article can be found in the online version, at DOI: 10.1016/j.thorsurg.2010.06.006.

REFERENCES

1. Gangolphe L. Enorme enchondrome de la fourchette sternale. Lyon Chir 1909;2:112 [in French].
2. Cotton BH, Paulsen GA, Dykes J. Prosthesis following excision of chest wall tumors. J Thorac Surg 1956;31(1):45–59.
3. Usher FC, Wallace S. Tissue reaction to plastics; a comparison of nylon, orlon, dacron, teflon, and marlex. AMA Arch Surg 1958;76(6):997–9.
4. Graham J, Usher FC, Perry JL, et al. Marlex mesh as a prosthesis in the repair of thoracic wall defects. Ann Surg 1960;151(4):469–79.
5. Le Roux BT, Shama DM. Resection of tumors of the chest wall. Curr Probl Surg 1983;20(6):345–86.

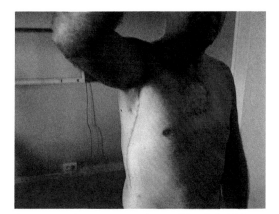

Fig. 10. Final cosmetic results. En bloc full-thickness chest wall resection involving the upper aspect of the sternum for a soft tissue sarcoma. Chest wall stabilization required a one-stage bridging osteosynthesis covered with a right latissimus dorsi transposition and free thin split-thickness skin graft.

6. McCormack P, Bains MS, Beattie EJ Jr, et al. New trends in skeletal reconstruction after resection of chest wall tumors. Ann Thorac Surg 1981;31(1):45–52.

7. Lardinois D, Müller M, Furrer M, et al. Functional assessment of chest wall integrity after methylmethacrylate reconstruction. Ann Thorac Surg 2000; 69(3):919–23.

8. Dahan M, Brouchet L, Berjaud J, et al. Chirurgie des tumeurs de la paroi thoracique. Ann Chir Plast Esthet 2003;48(2):93–8 [in French].

9. Borrelly J, Grosdidier G, Boileau S, et al. Chirurgie plastique de la paroi thoracique (déformations et tumeurs) a l'aide de l'attelle-agrafe à glissières. Ann Chir Plast Esthet 1990;35(1):57–61 [in French].

10. Coonar AS, Qureshi N, Smith I, et al. A novel titanium rib bridge system for chest wall reconstruction. Ann Thorac Surg 2009;87(5):e46–8.

11. Voss B, Bauernschmitt R, Brockmann G, et al. Osteosynthetic thoracic stabilization after complete resection of the sternum. Eur J Cardiothorac Surg 2007;32(2):391–3.

12. Hamad AM, Marulli G, Bulf R, et al. Titanium plates support for chest wall reconstruction with Gore-Tex dual mesh after sternochondral resection. Eur J Cardiothorac Surg 2009;36(4):779–80.

13. Iarussi T, Pardolesi A, Camplese P, et al. Composite chest wall reconstruction using titanium plates and mesh preserves chest wall function. J Thorac Cardiovasc Surg 2010;140(2):476–7.

14. Pedersen TA, Pilegaard HK. Reconstruction of the thorax with Ley prosthesis after resection of the sternum. Ann Thorac Surg 2009;87:e31–3.

15. Watanabe A, Watanabe T, Obama T, et al. New material for reconstruction of the anterior chest wall, including the sternum. J Thorac Cardiovasc Surg 2003;126(4):1212–4.

16. Tanaka H, Yukioka T, Yamaguti Y, et al. Surgical stabilization of internal pneumatic stabilization? A prospective randomized study of management of severe flail chest patients. J Trauma 2002;52(4):727–32.

17. Deschamps C, Tirnaksiz BM, Darbandi R, et al. Early and long-term results of prosthetic chest wall reconstruction. J Thorac Cardiovasc Surg 1999;117(3): 588–91.

18. Mansour KA, Thourani VH, Losken A, et al. Chest wall resections and reconstruction: a 25-year experience. Ann Thorac Surg 2002;73(6):1720–5.

19. Weyant MJ, Bains MS, Venkatraman E, et al. Results of chest wall resection and reconstruction with and without rigid prosthesis. Ann Thorac Surg 2006;81(1):279–85.

20. Daigeler A, Druecke D, Hakimi M, et al. Reconstruction of the thoracic wall-long-term follow-up including pulmonary function tests. Langenbecks Arch Surg 2009;394(4):705–15.

21. Chapelier AR, Missana MC, Couturaud B, et al. Sternal resection and reconstruction for primary malignant tumors. Ann Thorac Surg 2004;77(3):1001–6.

Overview on Current and Future Materials for Chest Wall Reconstruction

Gaetano Rocco, MD, FRCSEd, FETCS, FCCP*

KEYWORDS

- Chest wall reconstruction • Prosthesis • New materials

The focus of this article is on the new materials available to thoracic surgeons for the reconstruction of chest wall defects. Each surgeon is called to select the best reconstructive strategy based on the disease for which the resection is needed, the possible involvement of adjacent structures, the availability of professional colleagues for multidisciplinary involvement, and the preferred (or available) material for full or partial thickness reconstruction. It is emphasized that most of the time-honored materials for chest wall reconstruction described in the literature are still valuable inasmuch as they provide excellent coverage of inner organs by ensuring, at the same time, sufficient structural stability.[1-5] Nowadays, the real issue in chest wall reconstruction may ensue, as an example, from reiterated recurrences of primary chest wall tumors requiring several redo resections with possible concurrent involvement of the sternum.[6] Likewise, extensive and deep burns associated to multifocal fractures of the anterior ribs may demand an immediate reconstructive solution in the survivor.

In the current issue of the *Thoracic Surgery Clinics*, several contributors have described the use of either time-honored materials in combination with or independently used reconstruction compounds.[1-5] Today, complex chest wall reconstructions are performed by resorting to composite materials. Many of them result from a technological update of old concepts.[7,8] Recently, cryopreserved bony homografts have added a suitable option for minor and major reconstructive procedures with reduced morbidity and optimal structural configuration.[6,9]

THE CONCEPT OF A PROSTHESIS TO STABILIZE AND PROVIDE COVERAGE

Methylmethacrylate meshes or sandwiches, polytetrafluoroethylene (PTFE) or polypropylene patches, and polyglactin meshes belong to the routine thoracic surgical armamentarium, and the pitfalls and advantages of their use have been extensively described.[1-5] Nevertheless, the quest for the ideal material is not over, and the reason resides in

The user-friendliness in the placement and the adaptation to the chest wall defect to preserve function and cosmesis

The complexity of the immunogenicity reaction evoked in the host by the foreign material with the perspective incorporation of the prosthesis

The attendant risk for infection

The medium to long term of mechanical failure of the prosthesis

The possibility for the prosthesis to serve as marker for future reference in the event of resection for tumors with a potential for early recurrence.[1-6]

Moreover, a common denominator of all prostheses is the need for coverage with viable myocutaneous layers. Various flaps are available in the clinical practice to cover defects in the chest,[10]

Department of Thoracic Surgery and Oncology, Division of Thoracic Surgery, National Cancer Institute, Pascale Foundation, Naples, Italy
* Corresponding author. Via Terminio 1, 83028 Serino, Avellino, Italy.
E-mail address: Gaetano.Rocco@btopenworld.com

Thorac Surg Clin 20 (2010) 559–562
doi:10.1016/j.thorsurg.2010.06.005
1547-4127/10/$ – see front matter © 2010 Elsevier Inc. All rights reserved.

and these usually are used in primary operations mandating creative solutions[11,12] for subsequent reconstruction of the superficial layers. A theoretically appealing alternative should be to use a stabilizing and covering material that would not need a myocutaneous flap interposition. In the setting of replacing the sternum, the use of omentum to wrap the reconstructive material is advisable for its wide availability and the plastic properties well known to thoracic surgeons.[6]

THE ADAPTATION OF OLD CONCEPTS TO NEW MATERIALS

The restoration of the continuity of the body of resected ribs recently has been addressed by the application of clips or plates along the same lines as the stabilization of chest wall after multifocal fractures, yielding paradoxic chest wall movement and respiratory failure. Two different mechanical models of titanium clips and plates are available.[8,13–15] The first design recalls the time-honored Judet and Sanchez-LLoret plates inasmuch as these clips, available in different sizes, present claw-like projections, enabling the surgeon to adjust them tightly across the costal borders following elevation of the intercostal muscle and neurovascular pedicles (Stratos, Medexpert, Heitersheim, Germany).[8,13] In addition, bars can be connected to the clips by crimping; by an appropriate leverage mechanism, longer bars can be adjusted to stabilize the anterior chest wall after sternal resection. As a rule, additional materials (ie, PTFE) are applied for visceral coverage and structural support.[8]

An alternative and innovative fixation system design involves moldable titanium multiholed plates (Synthes, Solothurn, Switzerland) accommodating screws of different lengths to be drilled in the ribs or the sternum.[14,15] Several reports of the effectiveness of this system in providing stabilization after sternal resection have been published in the recent literature.[14,15] In addition, these plates have been used for chest wall reconstruction following sternal resection along with PTFE patches.[15] In this setting, there is a renewed interest toward the application for coverage and stabilization of sternal defects of shield-shaped titanium prosthesis (Ley prosthesis[16]), which has proven to successfully bridge sternal dehiscences after cardiac surgical procedures.[17]

A hydroxyapatite–tricalcium phosphate compound (ie, ceramic), shaped to morphologically and functionally replace the sternum, has been proposed for its user-friendly application, osteoconductivity, biomechanical resilience, and resistance to infections.[18] Although the elevated costs may prevent a more widespread clinical use of such ceramic implants, the attention of researchers investigating the possibility of deriving new reconstructive materials somehow revolves around hydroxyapatite scaffolds.

THE USE OF CRYOPRESERVED HOMOGRAFTS

A potentially inexhaustible source of biomaterials for chest wall reconstruction is the human cadaver.[19] Pioneered by orthopedic surgeons to fill bony defects and restore structural continuity,[20] the use of cryopreserved homografts has recently been successfully introduced in the thoracic surgical clinical practice.[6,9] Major advantages in using cryopreserved bony homografts include reduced immunogenicity, resistance to viral infection, and improved incorporation into the host environment due to revascularization and cellular repopulation.[6,21,22] Cadaveric homografts also fit in the geometric configuration of the chest wall, thereby enhancing the chances of functional preservation even in the event of use in combination with other materials for complex reconstructive efforts where multiple strategies and materials may be needed.[6,9]

THE PERSPECTIVES OF BIOMIMESIS APPLIED TO CLINICAL PRACTICE

The chest wall structure is composed of myocutaneous and fascial layers superimposed on an osteotendinous cage. Accordingly, the two major problems the thoracic surgeon is faced with when planning chest wall reconstruction will concern either the myocutaneous component alone or in association with the bony one. Potentially, as Metcalfe and Ferguson suggested, all skin layers could be replaced using a combination of "biomaterials, wound healing, embryonic development, stem cells and regeneration."[23] As an example, significant skin defects have been successfully covered with processed cadaveric skin or allogeneic neonatal fibroblasts.[23] In the last decade, collagen bioprostheses have increasingly polarized the attention of investigators aiming at replacing the myocutaneous defect of the breast and the abdominal wall.[23–26] Distinctive features of these biologic materials include resistance to infection, fibrovascular incorporation within the host surrounding structures, and avoidance of dense visceral adhesions.[23] Moreover, the use of bioprostheses is not related to any donor site morbidity. Both human and porcine acellular biologic collagen meshes have been proposed to establish continuity of coverage in deep defects in adjunct to myocutaneous flaps in the process of repair of complex abdominal wall defects.[23] The use of commercially available dermocutaneous substitutes presents common pitfalls, which may be significant when considering their use on the chest wall, ranging from fragility of coverage to antigenicity leading to graft rejection.[23] Nevertheless, processed cadaveric cutaneous allografts have been used to generate tissue expansion aimed at creating a wide enough pocket to accommodate a breast prosthesis following mastectomy with excellent short- and medium-term results.[27] Overall, viability of cadaveric allografts has been confirmed in the event of irradiated or infected breasts.[28] The use of acellular dermal matrix in conjunction with muscle flap for chest wall reconstruction has been described by Cothren and colleagues.[29] The advantageous features of cadaveric dermal substitutes have led to their experimental use in the rabbit model to cover lateral chest wall defects.[30] Interestingly, the resilience to rupture of the dermal substitutes was greater than PTFE and contralateral intact chest wall.[30]

BIODEGRADABLE MATERIALS FOR RIB SUBSTITUTES

Biodegradable compounds, like collagen-coated polydioxanone and polycaprolactone struts reinforced by chitin fiber, have been recently investigated as materials to construct absorbable meshes to cover chest wall defects.[31] The combination of polydioxanone mesh, demineralized bone, and bone marrow stromal cells has been successfully used in an animal model to replace ribs and reconstruct a relatively small chest wall defect.[32] A striking property of this substitute composite resided in the affinity of geometric and biomechanical features compared with the animal ribs.[32] Osteogenic cells cultured in scaffolds made of polycaprolactone (a biodegradable polymer) incorporating fragmented hydroxyapatite have demonstrated signs of osteogenic differentiation both in vitro and in vivo.[33] In addition, segments of bone have been generated through collagen–hydroxyapatite scaffolds and autologous platelet-enriched plasma.[34] Recently, hydroxyapatite bone scaffolds have been obtained from highly porous pine and rattan wood[35] through a five-step process including

> Pyrolysis (at 1000°C, creating carbon templates)
> Carburization (ie, transformation into calcium carbides through vapor and liquid-phase infiltration)
> Oxidation (ie, transformation into calcium oxide templates)

> Carbonation (ie, adding CO_2 through fluxing or compressing the gas through a furnace or a hydrothermal reactor)
> Phosphatization (ie, transformation of calcium carbonate templates into porous hydroxyapatite ceramics by adding KH_2PO_4).[35]

The distinctive feature of this model is to offer a structure characterized by a tubular, multilevel organization ideal for revascularization, osteogenesis, and biomechanical resilience.[35]

SUMMARY

New materials and the adaptation of new concepts to time-honored compounds have contributed to expand the technical options for chest wall reconstruction. The possibility of deriving biocompatible substitutes for all chest wall layers from previously unimaginable and potentially inexhaustible sources discloses unprecedented technological horizons.

REFERENCES

1. Deschamps C, Tirnaksiz BM, Darbandi R, et al. Early and long-term results of prosthetic chest wall reconstruction. J Thorac Cardiovasc Surg 1999;117: 588–91.
2. Mansour KA, Thourani VH, Losken A, et al. Chest wall resections and reconstruction: a 25-year experience. Ann Thorac Surg 2002;73:1720–5.
3. Lardinois D, Müller M, Furrer M, et al. Functional assessment of chest wall integrity after methylmethacrylate reconstruction. Ann Thorac Surg 2000; 69:919–23.
4. Weyant MJ, Bains MS, Venkatraman E, et al. Results of chest wall resection and reconstruction with and without rigid prosthesis. Ann Thorac Surg 2006;81: 279–85.
5. Chapelier AR, Missana MC, Couturaud B, et al. Sternal resection and reconstruction for primary malignant tumors. Ann Thorac Surg 2004;77: 1001–6.
6. Rocco G, Fazioli F, Scognamiglio F, et al. The combination of multiple materials in the creation of an artificial anterior chest cage after extensive demolition for recurrent chondrosarcoma. J Thorac Cardiovasc Surg 2007;133:1112–4.
7. Voss B, Bauernschmitt R, Brockmann G, et al. Osteosynthetic thoracic stabilization after complete resection of the sternum. Eur J Cardiothorac Surg 2007;32:391–3.
8. Coonar AS, Qureshi N, Smith I, et al. A novel titanium rib bridge system for chest wall reconstruction. Ann Thorac Surg 2009;87:e46–8.
9. Marulli G, Hamad AM, Cogliati E, et al. Allograft sternochondral replacement after resection of large

sternal chondrosarcoma. J Thorac Cardiovasc Surg 2010;139:e69–70.

10. Arnold PG, Pairolero PC. Chest-wall reconstruction: an account of 500 consecutive patients. Plast Reconstr Surg 1996;98:804–10.

11. Itano H, Andou A, Date H, et al. Chest wall reconstruction with perforator flaps after wide full-thickness resection. J Thorac Cardiovasc Surg 2006;132:e13–4.

12. Rocco G, Scognamiglio F, Fazioli F, et al. V-Y latissimus dorsi flap for coverage of anterior chest wall defects after resection of recurrent chest wall chondrosarcoma. J Thorac Cardiovasc Surg 2009;138:1242–3.

13. Pompili C, Brunelli A, Xiume' F, et al. Chest wall reconstruction with a titanium rib bridge for posttraumatic parietal hernia. Eur J Cardiothorac Surg 2010;37:737.

14. Voss B, Bauernschmitt R, Will A, et al. Sternal reconstruction with titanium plates in complicated sternal dehiscence. Eur J Cardiothorac Surg 2008;34:139–45.

15. Hamad AM, Marulli G, Bulf R, et al. Titanium plates support for chest wall reconstruction with Gore-Tex dual mesh after sternochondral resection. Eur J Cardiothorac Surg 2009;36:779–80.

16. Astudillo R, Vaage J, Myhre U, et al. Fewer reoperations and shorter stay in the cardiac surgical ward when stabilising the sternum with the Ley prosthesis in post-operative mediastinitis. Eur J Cardiothorac Surg 2001;20:133–9.

17. Pedersen TAL, Pilegaard HK. Reconstruction of the thorax with Ley prosthesis after resection of the sternum. Ann Thorac Surg 2009;87:e31–3.

18. Watanabe A, Watanabe T, Obama T, et al. New material for reconstruction of the anterior chest wall, including the sternum. J Thorac Cardiovasc Surg 2003;126:1212–4.

19. Garcia-Tutor E, Yeste L, Murillo J, et al. Chest wall reconstruction using iliac bone allografts and muscle flaps. Ann Plast Surg 2004;52:54–60.

20. Simpson D, Kakarala G, Hampson K, et al. Viable cells survive in fresh frozen human bone allografts. Acta Orthop 2007;78:26–30.

21. Judas F, Rosa S, Teixeira L, et al. Chondrocyte viability in fresh and frozen large human osteochondral allografts: effect of cryoprotective agents. Transplant Proc 2007;39:2531–4.

22. Tomford WW, Mankin HJ, Friedlaender GE, et al. Methods of banking bone and cartilage for allograft transplantation. Orthop Clin North Am 1987;18:241–7.

23. Metcalfe AD, Ferguson MWJ. Tissue engineering in the replacement of skin:the crossroads of biomaterials, wound healing, embryonic development, stem cells and regeneration. J R Soc Interface 2007;4:413–37.

24. Butler CE. The role of bioprosthetics in abdominal wall reconstruction. Clin Plast Surg 2006;33:199–211.

25. Chavarriaga LF, Lin E, Losken A, et al. Management of complex abdominal wall defects using acellular porcine dermal collagen. Am Surg 2010;76:96–100.

26. Palao R, Gómez P, Huguet P. Burned breast reconstructive surgery with Integra dermal regeneration template. Br J Plast Surg 2003;56:252–9.

27. Bindingnavele V, Gaon M, Ota KS, et al. Use of acellular cadaveric dermis and tissue expansion in postmastectomy breast reconstruction. J Plast Reconstr Aesthet Surg. 2007;60:1214–8.

28. Nahabedian MY. AlloDerm performance in the setting of prosthetic breast surgery, infection, and irradiation. Plast Reconstr Surg 2009;124:1743–53.

29. Cothren CC, Gallego K, Anderson ED, et al. Chest wall reconstruction with acellular dermal matrix (AlloDerm) and a latissimus muscle flap. Plast Reconstr Surg 2004;114:1015–7.

30. Holton LH, Chung T, Silverman RP, et al. Comparison of acellular dermal matrix and synthetic mesh for lateral chest wall reconstruction in a rabbit model. Plast Reconstr Surg 2007;119:1238–46.

31. Qin X, Tang H, Xu Z, et al. Chest wall reconstruction with two types of biodegradable polymer prostheses in dogs. Eur J Cardiothorac Surg 2008;34:870–4.

32. Tang H, Xu Z, Qin X, et al. Chest wall reconstruction in a canine model using polydioxanone mesh, demineralized bone matrix and bone marrow stromal cells. Biomaterials 2009;30:3224–33.

33. Chuenjitkuntaworn B, Inrung W, Damrongsri D, et al. Polycaprolactone/hydroxyapatite composite scaffolds: Preparation, characterization, and in vitro and in vivo biological responses of human primary bone cells. J Biomed Mater Res A 2010;94:241–51.

34. Chang SH, Hsu YM, Wang YJ, et al. Fabrication of pre-determined shape of bone segment with collagen-hydroxyapatite scaffold and autogenous platelet-rich plasma. J Mater Sci Mater Med 2009;20:23–31.

35. Tampieri A, Sprio S, Ruffini A, et al. From wood to bone: multi-step process to convert wood hierarchical structures into biomimetic hydroxyapatite scaffolds for bone tissue engineering. J Mater Chem 2009;19:4973–80.

Pectus Carinatum

Francis Robicsek, MD, PhD*, Larry T. Watts, MD

KEYWORDS
- Pectus carinatum • Chest deformity • Pouter pigeon breast
- Surgical management

The chest becomes sharply pointed and not broad and becomes affected with difficulty in breathing and hoarseness.

Hippocrates[1]

Pectus carinatum or keel chest is a spectrum of progressive inborn anomalies of the anterior chest wall, named after the keel (carina) of ancient Roman ships. It defines a wide spectrum of inborn protrusion anomalies of the sternum and/or the adjacent costal cartilages.[2]

Pectus carinatum is seen less frequently than pectus excavatum anomalies and occurs in about 0.06% of all live births.[3] More recent studies using computed tomography suggest that milder forms of the anomaly are more frequent and occur in about 2% of children, whereas asymmetrical prominence of costal cartilages occur in 5% of children. Men are 4 times more frequently affected, and one-third of the patients have a family history of some type of anterior chest deformity.[4,5]

Although the pathophysiology of pectus carinatum is not fully known, it is the generally accepted view that in both pectus excavatum and carinatum, the cause is not the sternum but the genetically[6] defective elongated cartilages. If the cartilages push the sternum forward by their accelerated growth, pectus carinatum develops; if they dislocate the sternum posteriorly, it results in pectus excavatum.[7] Other proposed causes include anomalous development of the diaphragm and premature fusion of the sternal growth centers.[8]

Pectus carinatum is often associated with various conditions, notably Marfan disease, homocystinuria, prune belly, Morquio syndrome, osteogenesis imperfecta, Noonan syndrome, and mitral valve prolapse.[9,10] The suggestion that there is also a strong link with congenital heart disease[8] may be misleading. A wide variety of congenital heart anomalies result in right ventricular hypertrophy, which may cause bulging of the precordium and gives the appearance of keel chest (pseudo pectus carinatum). Overzealous pectus excavatum repair may result in iatrogenic pectus carinatum.[9,10] Such a situation may develop if forward-convex rigid bars, such as those used in the Nuss procedure, are applied. A heretofore unknown form of iatrogenic pectus condition, reactive pectus carinatum, was recently described and attributed to fibroelastic changes of the sternum and the costal cartilages stimulated by implanted metal bars.[11]

Symmetric pectus carinatum is the condition that fits best with the term keel chest. The sternum broadly arches forward, often with mild relative depression of the costal cartilages, which may accentuate the sternal prominence.[12] Symmetric pectus carinatum has 2 common varieties: in one, the xyphoid process meets the lower end of the sternum in a forward 90° angle (**Fig. 1**) and in the other, the xyphoid remains in a straight continuation of the sternal axis.

In a less frequently seen symmetric anomaly, the sternal prominence is moderate or absent, but there is a bilateral protruding ridge of costal cartilages (**Fig. 2**).

Asymmetrical varieties of pectus carinatum are numerous. In most cases the sternum is tilted, usually toward the right. In that form, the costal cartilages are prominent on one side and the sternum is tilted toward the sunken contralateral side. This deformity may be best called combined carinatum and excavatum (**Fig. 3**).

Department of Thoracic and Cardiovascular Surgery, Sanger Heart and Vascular Institute, Carolinas Medical Center, 1001 Blythe Boulevard, Suite 300, Charlotte, NC 28203, USA
* Corresponding author.
E-mail address: francis.robicsek@carolinashealthcare.org

Thorac Surg Clin 20 (2010) 563–574
doi:10.1016/j.thorsurg.2010.07.007

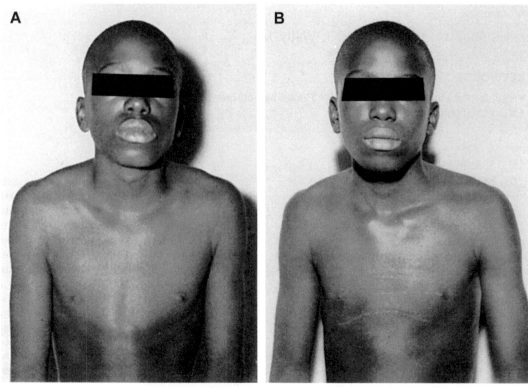

Fig. 1. Typical pectus carinatum deformity with xyphoid angulation before (*A*) and after (*B*) surgical repair. (*From* Robicsek F. Surgical treatment of pectus carinatum. Chest Surg Clin N Am 2000;10:357–76.)

In some patients, there is only an individual prominence of a single costal cartilage, whereas in others with the so-called cartilaginous ridges, there is a whole row of cartilages that protrude parallel to the normally positioned sternum (**Fig. 4**).

In pouter pigeon breast (chondromanubrial prominence with chondrogladiolar depression),

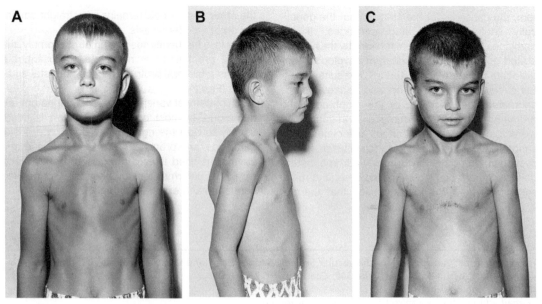

Fig. 2. Pectus carinatum with bilateral protrusion of the costal cartilages before (*A*) and after (*B, C*) surgical repair.

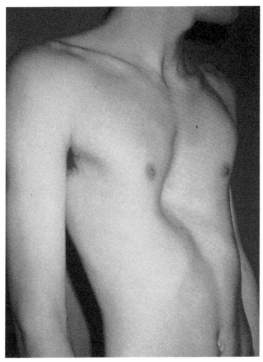

Fig. 3. Combination of pectus carinatum and excavatum.

there is significant thickening and protrusion of a thickened manubrium. The anomaly is usually associated with moderate to severe depression of the sternal body (gladiolus) (**Fig. 5**).

Unlike pectus excavatum, the extent of symmetric pectus carinatum is usually appreciated later in life. The infantile protruding belly recedes during early puberty and makes the prominence of the precordium more apparent. Because carinatum deformities are more difficult to conceal with clothing or posture, they are more likely to cause social withdrawal and poor self-perception. Thus, cosmesis in pectus carinatum is more of an issue than it is in pectus excavatum of comparable severity.

Corrective surgery in pectus carinatum is performed not only for cosmetic reasons but also for alleviating existing or preventing future cardiopulmonary and postural abnormalities. Physiologic testing at rest usually yields normal values; however, cardiac and pulmonary function may be adversely affected under exercise conditions. By the time the patients reach adolescence, many complain of decreased endurance and exertional dyspnea. This condition is believed to be caused by fixed anteroposterior diameter with consequential lowered pulmonary compliance, decreased respiratory movements of the chest wall, development of emphysematous changes, and frequent respiratory tract infections.[13-15]

Different opinions have been expressed on the optimum time for surgery. The authors do not share the opinion of those[16] who suggest that the repair of pectus deformities should be delayed until puberty or later because of the danger of restricting the development of the juvenile thorax. If the intervention is performed properly, that is, if attention is given to preserve the cartilaginous growth centers, the repair of pectus deformities may be safely performed in the young child.[17-20] In adult patients, the operation is more complex and the functional and psychological changes are more severe. Good cosmetic results with marked improvement in endurance, dyspnea, and exercise may still be achieved for repair in adulthood.[4]

In his first report on surgical repair of the keel chest, Ravitch[21] called it "an unusual sternal deformity with cardiac symptoms" that should be treated with sternal osteotomy and cartilaginous resection. About the same time, Lester[2] developed a more radical procedure consisting not only of bilateral resection of the protuberant cartilages but also of subperiosteal removal of the corresponding portion of the sternum. Ravitch[21] later modified his original procedure by performing a transverse sternotomy and placing perichondrial reefing sutures to secure the corrected position of the sternum. Chin[22] in 1957 attempted to correct keel chest by transferring the mobilized xyphoid process into an anterior midsternal slot. In 1963,[23-25] the authors introduced the method described later, which has been applied successfully for the repair of pectus carinatum with minor modifications throughout the past 4 decades.[26-34]

THE AUTHORS' TECHNIQUE OF SYMMETRIC PECTUS CARINATUM REPAIR

A 4- to 5-cm—long upward-convex incision centered at the level of the sternoxyphoid junction is made. By retracting the skin and subcutaneous tissue in a single flap, the sternum and the pectoralis fascia are exposed.

Using electrocautery, the pectoralis major muscles are detached from the sternum then bilaterally retracted, and the involved portion of the sternum and respective costal cartilages are exposed. The authors have found that special methods to facilitate adequate exposure through a small skin incision, such as the application of video camera and CO_2 insufflation, have been[35,36] unnecessary.

Restoration of the chest to a normal shape begins with a conservative subperichondrial

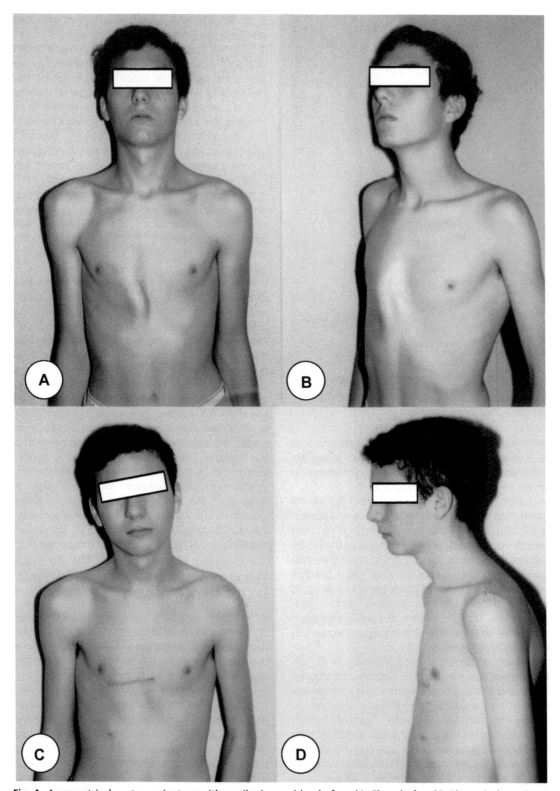

Fig. 4. Asymmetrical pectus carinatum with cartilaginous ridge before (*A, B*) and after (*C, D*) surgical repair.

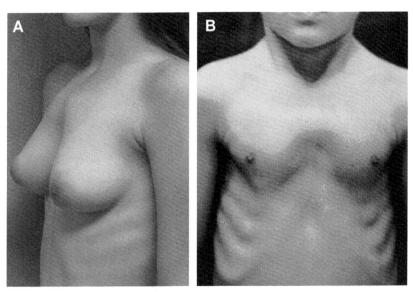

Fig. 5. Pouter pigeon chest types A (*A*) and B (*B*).

resection of the protruding cartilages. This resection is seldom performed above the fourth and practically never above the third rib. The lateral extent of the resection increases as the procedure is carried downward. Care is exerted to preserve the growth potentials of the juvenile thorax by leaving the underlying perichondrium and preserving the growth centers of the cartilages at the costochondral junction. Resection of the bony portion of ribs may become necessary in adults. The xyphoid process is detached from the sternum. Using a wide osteotome, a linear transverse sternal osteotomy is done at the level of the interspace above the uppermost resected costal cartilage. The depth of the osteotomy should reach, but not cross, the posterior sternal lamina. The sternal protrusion is now corrected by manual green-branch fracturing of the sternum at the osteotomy site and pressing it posteriorly. A 3- to 4-cm portion of the sternum is resected from the lower end, and using 2-0 nonabsorbable sutures the previously disconnected xyphoid process is reattached to the lower sternal stump. This way the traction of the rectus abdominis muscles is transmitted to the sternum and keeps it in a corrected position (**Fig. 6**). This new position of the sternum is further reinforced by uniting the detached edges of the pectoralis major muscles presternally. This maneuver not only helps to restrain the sternum but also provides a smooth presternal padding and enhances bony healing (**Fig. 7**).[37] A small suction catheter is left in the wound for 24 hours and the incision is closed in 2 layers using fine filaments. A thick dressing is applied firmly over the wound and changed after

the drain is removed. Thereafter, the dressing need not be applied with pressure. Postoperative management may be enhanced by the routine use of indwelling epidural catheter placed at the time of surgery. In the authors' practice, this strategy significantly reduced the amount of narcotics required and allowed earlier mobilization. Patients are recommended to avoid strenuous activity for 3 to 6 months, especially if it involves contact sports.

Although this technique contains elements of the original operations of Lester[2] and Ravitch,[21] it differs from theirs in several respects such as avoiding wide exposure and introducing sternal shortening and xyphoid reattachment. Also, in this technique, avoidance of use of rods or plates for any form of pectus repairs (carinatum or excavatum) is strongly emphasized. Use of rods or plates is not only unnecessary and in many respects dangerous but also the need for reoperation for their removal is illogical.

Postoperative results of pectus carinatum are measured in terms of both cosmesis and function. Reflecting on the differences in the postoperative results of pectus carinatum and excavatum repair, one may expect that the various aspects in surgical engineering in the correction of these 2 chest deformities should be considered. The repair of pectus excavatum is frequently confronted with flat-chested asthenic individuals, several with Marfan disease, in whom elevating the anterior chest wall to a desired level and keeping it in a permanently corrected position may be fraught with difficulties. The surgeon may have to accept less than ideal postoperative

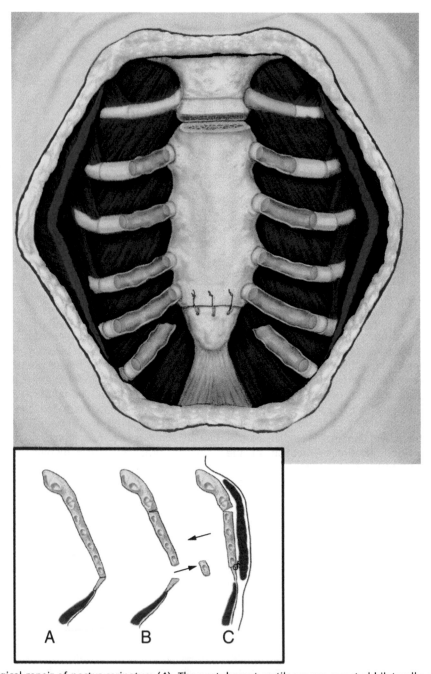

Fig. 6. Surgical repair of pectus carinatum (*A*). The protuberant cartilages are resected bilaterally, a transverse sternotomy is done at the upper level of the deformity, a portion of the lower sternum is resected (*arrows*), (*B*) and the xyphoid process is reattached (*C*). (*From* Robicsek F. Surgical treatment of pectus carinatum. Chest Surg Clin N Am 2000;10:357–76.)

results. In pectus carinatum, the repair encompasses properly positioning the sternum and the removal of protruding tissues. Less than excellent results are unacceptable.

Studies on functional changes after pectus carinatum repair are scarce and controversial. While some observed marked improvement in patients with preoperatively reduced stamina and in vital capacity, others found no differences in pre- and postoperative work tolerance.[37,38] This contradiction is even more prevalent in patients with carinatum than excavatum anomalies.

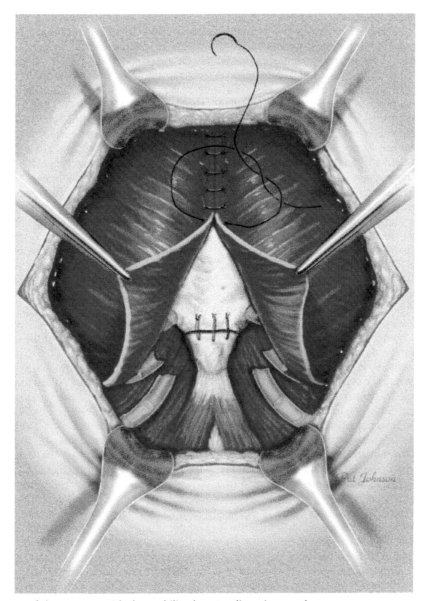

Fig. 7. Coverage of the sternum with the mobilized pectoralis major muscles.

In patients with lateral or asymmetrical pectus carinatum, the pinnacle of the protrusion is usually the costochondral junction with the bony rib bending in anteriorly and the cartilages in the posterior direction.[39] While in some cases only 1 or 2 ribs are involved, in most patients 3 or more ribs are protruding creating a ridge. Surgical treatment consists of simple excision of the protuberant ribs. Exposure of unilateral deformities, especially in female patients, may be obtained through a short submammary incision. If a ridge composed of 4 or more cartilages needs to be excised, it is advisable to remove short parasternal segments of the

contralateral cartilages as well, to prevent the flipping of the sternum by the retained ribs.

Pouter pigeon breast, also called as Currarino-Silverman syndrome[40] or chondrogladiolar prominence with chondrosternal depression, is characterized by the protrusion of the abnormally thick sternal manubrium and the C-shaped backward-arching sternal body. The xyphoid process points slightly anteriorly, which further exaggerates the sunken appearance of the mesosternum. The condition is attributed to premature fusion or absence of the sternal ossification centers,[40] and this is the chest deformity that is most often associated with congenital heart disease. The clinical symptoms of pigeon breast overlap those of other varieties of pectus carinatum. Respiratory consequences are rare and seem to be caused by the caudal depression rather than the manubrial prominence. Because of the manubrial prominence, the anomaly is difficult to conceal and is often accompanied with severe psychological consequences.

The first operation for pouter pigeon breast was performed by Ravitch[21] in 1952. The procedure consisted of removing the deformed cartilages and performing 2 transverse sternal osteotomies: one in the area of prominence and the other in the midportion of the sternal body (Ravitch 1952). The manubrium was left intact.

In the authors' technique of pouter pigeon breast repair,[19,23,26,28,31,41] the skin incision is made somewhat higher than applied in symmetric carinatum repair. Depending on the morphology of the anomaly, the sternum is surgically modified in one of the following ways:

In type A of pouter pigeon breast, in which the depression of the sternal body is only moderate, the abnormal anatomy is dominated by the protrusion of the thickened manubrium and the 2 adjacent cartilages. The repair is limited only to the manubrial area. First, the protruding portion of the second and third costal cartilages is resected. A deep transverse groove is then gauged into the lower end of the manubrial prominence to allow the proper positioning of a wide osteotome to chisel off the thickness of the anterior portion of the manubrium (**Fig. 8**).

In type B anomaly, the sternal body is significantly depressed. In such cases, in addition to the procedure described earlier for type A variety, the depressed sternal body is treated similar to a primary pectus excavatum repair.[42] The pectoralis muscles are detached bilaterally, and a transverse-wedge sternotomy is made at the upper level of the depression. The deformed costal cartilages are subperichondrially resected. The sternum is then freed of its mediastinal and intercostal attachments, green-branch fractured, bent forward, and a sheet of Marlex mesh (C. R. Bard, Inc, Salt Lake City, UT, USA) is placed under it. The mesh is anchored in a stretched-tight position with nonabsorbable sutures to the lateral stumps of the resected costal cartilages. To ensure proper wound drainage, the right pleural cavity is deliberately entered and widely connected with the retrosternal space and drained through an intercostal catheter. The previously detached edges of the pectoralis major muscles are united presternally (see **Fig. 7**).

Occasionally, patients present themselves with protrusion deformities, best described as a combination of pectus carinatum and excavatum. In such cases, one side of the anterior chest wall, usually the left, is sunken and the contralateral side is protuberant. The sternum is rotated toward the depressed side (**Fig. 9**).

The initial portion of the repair (ie, exposure of the sternum, transverse osteotomy, detachment of the xyphoid process, and the subperichondrial resection of the involved cartilages) is identical with the method described earlier for the correction of the symmetric keel chest. After that, however, the sternum is detached from the intercostal and pericardial tissues, green-branch fractured at the osteotomy site, and forcefully twisted toward the protuberant side into a normal horizontal position. This corrected position of the sternum is then secured by a "reversed Z" wire suture (see **Fig. 8**). A sheath of Marlex mesh is placed under the sternum and anchored in a stretched-on with heavy nonabsorbable sutures to the medial ends of the divided costal cartilages. The right pleural cavity is deliberately entered, connected widely with the retrosternal space, and drained with an intercostal catheter. The xyphoid process is left detached and the pectoralis major muscles are united presternally. After the closure of the skin, the shape of the chest is carefully reexamined. If any lumps or bumps are left, one should not hesitate to reopen the incision and make additional corrections.

Different forms of pectus carinatum are often associated with abnormalities of the spine, such as scoliosis, lordosis, and kyphosis. Depending on the situation, either the anterior (pectus carinatum) or the posterior anomaly (kyphosis) could be the primary component of deformed chest. The cause of these anomalies may be genetic or due to failure of vertebrae formation or segmentation.[27] Keel chest may also develop as a structural necessity. Whenever the spinal column shortens, it forces the anterior chest wall to bulge forward to achieve a comparable decrease of its vertical axis. Characteristically, patients with kyphosis-induced keel chest suffer the most significant cardiorespiratory changes; many of them die of cor pulmonale. As a rule, if a patient considered for surgical repair of pectus carinatum has significant spinal anomaly as well, an orthopedic specialist with special interest in juvenile diseases of the spine should be an integral part of both planning and treatment.[18,28]

With the ongoing pandemic of the so-called minimally invasive (Nuss and colleagues)[43] operation for pectus excavatum, it was expected that similar techniques will be applied to treat pectus

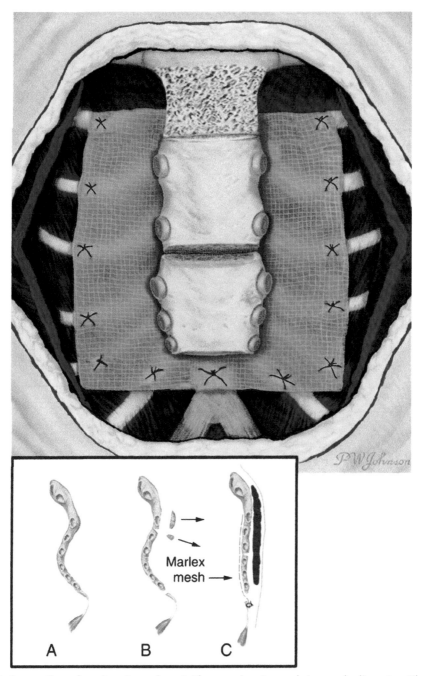

Fig. 8. Surgical correction of pouter pigeon breast. The prominent manubrium and adjacent cartilages are leveled off with an osteotome. If the sternal body is depressed (type B), the xyphoid process is detached, the respective cartilages are also resected, and the sternal axis is corrected with 2 transverse sternal osteotomies and rested on a Marlex mesh sutured tout to the stumps of the resected cartilages. (*From* Robicsek F. Surgical treatment of pectus carinatum. Chest Surg Clin N Am 2000;10:357–76.)

carinatum as well. Abramson and colleagues[44] reported a novel method by which Nuss bars are applied outside the bony thorax in a subcutaneous or submuscular position to create lasting compression strong enough to remodel the keel chest to a normal shape. The bar is left in the patients for an excess of 2 years. After bar removal, the results in 10 out of 20 patients were labeled as excellent. Complications included infection, fracture and dislocation of the bar,

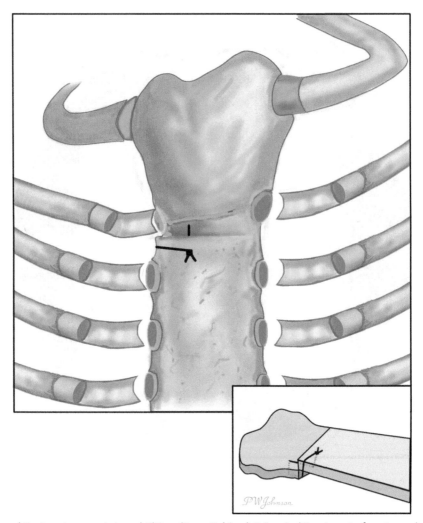

Fig. 9. Reversed Z suture to correct sternal tilting. (*From* Robicsek F. Surgical Treatment of pectus carinatum. Chest Surg Clin N Am 2000;10:357–76.)

chondral overgrowth requiring reoperation, conversion to conventional repair, and in several cases, adherence of the bar to the skin.

The same arguments may be raised against the Abramson operation designed to treat pectus carinatum as one may dispute the alleged merits of the minimally invasive Nuss procedure that is now widely in use to manage pectus excavatum. The limited-exposure open repair that is applied may be more justifiably defined as minimally invasive than the Nuss or the Abramson procedure. This repair has limited potential for serious and, occasionally, deadly complications that occur in the Nuss and Abramson repair. It neither leaves large steel bars in the body for years nor requires reoperations to remove them. In this ongoing

debate between open and closed repair of pectus anomalies, it is also emphasized that most open pectus operations radically differ from the Ravitch procedure,[27] which provided no reliable sternal stability, and was performed through large vertical exposures leaving long and unsightly scars. However, those who tout the advantages of the so-called minimally invasive interventions still uses the nonhomogenous group of patients operated with different types of classic or modified Ravitch procedures as a control group to which their novel intervention is compared. The authors suggest to eliminate the term modified Ravitch repair altogether, because nowadays there are so many procedures that may include some of the elements of the classical Ravitch operation but their general approach widely differs from it. It is also difficult to fathom as to why the Abramson technique, and especially the Nuss technique, which crosses through body cavities and leaves foot-long metal bars in the body up to several years, is called minimally invasive.

The latest development in this "do anything but do not leave any scars" trend is the method introduced by Kim and Idowu,[45] that is, the intrathoracic resection of the deformed ribs using thoracoscopic technology. So far it has been applied only for localized unilateral lesions. It requires the patient to wear an external compression binder for a year.

Although the general opinion certainly favors interventional treatment in different pectus carinatum modalities, compressive orthotic methods have also been recommended to treat milder cases of pectus carinatum.[46] In most of these studies, patient compliance in wearing compressive braces for extended periods has been poor.[47] Also, in several studies and in which favorable results were reported,[34] the investigators relied on satisfaction surveys or other subjective evaluations and not on objective anthropomorphic measurements. There has been no major study that has proved significant anatomic improvement induced by compressive brace treatment. As the general opinion stands today, nonsurgical treatment with exercise and casting has not been worthwhile, whereas surgical management is simple and successful.

SUMMARY

The proper requirements for the modern treatment of pectus carinatum include the following:

> Should be simple and swift
> Should not leave rigid foreign materials in the body
> Should not create a potential for serious complications
> Should provide uniformly excellent cosmetic and functional results
> Should not necessitate extended and frequent follow-up
> Should not require reintervention.

Nothing short of these requirements should be accepted.

REFERENCES

1. Hippocrates quote by Castile RG, Staats BA, Westbook PR. Symptomatic pectus deformities in 116 adults. Ann Surg 2002;236:304–14.

2. Lester CW. Pigeon breast (pectus carinatum) and other protrusion deformities of the chest of developmental origin. Ann Surg 1953;137:482–9.

3. Mielke CH, Winter RB. Pectus carinatum successfully treated with bracing: a case report. Int Orthop 1993;17:350–2.

4. Fonkalsrud EW, Bustorff-Silva J. Repair of pectus excavatum and carinatum in adults. Am J Surg 1999;177:121–4.

5. Welch KJ, Vos A. Surgical correction of pectus carinatum (pigeon breast). J Pediatr Surg 1973;8(5):659–67.

6. Fokin AA, Steuerwald NM, Ahrens WA, et al. Anatomical, histologic and genetic characteristics of congenital chest wall deformities. Semin Thorac Cardiovasc Surg 2009;21:44–57.

7. Robicsek F. Pectus excavatum and carinatum. In: Grillo HC, Austen WE, Wilkins EW, et al, editors. Current therapy in cardiac surgery. Toronto (Canada): BC Decker Inc; 1989. p. 87–90.

8. Harcke HT, Grissom LE, Lee MS, et al. Common congenital skeletal anomalies of the thorax. J Thorac Imaging 1986;1(4):1–6.

9. Hebra A, Swoveland B, Egbert M, et al. Outcome analysis of minimally invasive repair of pectus excavatum: review of 251 cases. J Pediatr Surg 2000;35:252–8.

10. Taybi H. Radiology of syndromes and metabolic disorders. Chicago: Ed: Year Book; 1983.

11. Swanson JW, Colombani PM. Reactive pectus carinatum in patients treated for pectus excavatum. J Pediatr Surg 2008;43:1468–73.

12. Ravitch MM. Operative treatment of congenital deformities of the chest. Am J Surg 1961;101:588–97.

13. Pickard LR, Tepas JJ, Shermeta DW, et al. Pectus carinatum. Results of surgical therapy. J Pediatr Surg 1979;14:228–30.

14. Castile RG, Staats BA, Westbrook PR. Symptomatic pectus deformities of the chest. Am Rev Respir Dis 1982;126:564–8.

15. Lam CR, Taber RE. Surgical treatment of pectus carinatum. Arch Surg 1971;103:191–4.

16. Haller JA, Colombani PM, Humphries CT, et al. Chest wall constriction after too extensive and too early operations for pectus excavatum. Ann Thorac Surg 1996;61:1618–25.

17. Robicsek F, Fokin AA. How not to do it: restrictive thoracic dystrophy after pectus excavatum repair. Interact Cardiovasc Thorac Surg 2004;3(4):566–8.

18. Robicsek F. Surgical treatment of pectus excavatum. In: Robicsek F, Faber LP, editors. Chest surgery clinics of North America, vol. 2. Philadelphia: W.B. Saunders Company; 2000. p. 277–96.

19. Robicsek F. Surgical treatment of pectus carinatum. In: Robicsek F, Faber LP, editors. Chest surgery clinics of North America, vol. 2. Philadelphia: W.B. Saunders Company; 2000. p. 357–76.

20. Robicsek F, Fokin A. How not to do it: restrictive thoracic dystrophy after pectus excavatum repair. Interact Cardiovasc Thorac Surg 2004;3:566—8.

21. Ravitch MM. Unusual sternal deformity with cardiac symptoms: operative correction. J Thorac Surg 1952;23:138.

22. Chin EF. Surgery of funnel chest and congenital sternal prominence. Br J Surg 1957;44:360.

23. Robicsek F, Sanger PW, Taylor FH, et al. The surgical treatment of chondrosternal prominence (pectus carinatum). J Thorac Cardiovasc Surg 1963;45:691—701.

24. Sanger PW, Robicsek F, Taylor FH. Surgical management of anterior chest deformities: a new technique and report of 153 operations without a death. Surgery 1960;48:510—21.

25. Sanger PW, Taylor FH, Robicsek F. Deformities of the anterior chest wall. Surg Gynecol Obstet 1963;116:515—22.

26. Robicsek F, Daugherty HK, Mullen DC, et al. Technical considerations in the surgical management of pectus excavatum and carinatum. Ann Thorac Surg 1974;18:549—64.

27. Robicsek F, Cook JW, Daugherty HK, et al. Pectus carinatum. J Thorac Cardiovasc Surg 1979;78:52—61.

28. Robicsek F. Congenital deformities of the anterior chest wall. In: Gellis SS, Kagan BM, editors. Current pediatric therapy. Philadelphia: W.B. Saunders; 1986. p. 413—4.

29. Robicsek F. Pectus carinatum. Tokyo: Published in the collected works of the International Thoracic Congress; 1988. p. 235—56.

30. Robicsek F. Surgical repair of pectus excavatum and carinatum deformities. J Cardiovasc Surg 1998;39(Suppl 1):155—9.

31. Robicsek F, Fokin A. Surgical correction of pectus excavatum and carinatum. J Cardiovasc Surg (Torino) 1999;40(5):725—31.

32. Robicsek F. Preface. Chest surgery clinics of North America. In: Robicsek F, Faber LP, editors. Chest surgery clinics of North America, vol. 2. Philadelphia: W.B. Saunders Company; 2000. p. xi.

33. Robicsek F, Fokin A, Watts L. Surgical treatment of anterior chest deformities. Controversy upon controversy. European Respiratory Society. Berlin, Germany. Eur Respir J 2008;32(52):497(E2834).

34. Robicsek F, Watts LT, Fokin AA. Surgical repair of pectus excavatum and carinatum. Semin Thorac Cardiovasc Surg 2009;21:64—75.

35. Schaarschmidt K, Kolberg-Schwerdt A, Lempe M, et al. New endoscopic minimal access pectus carinatum repair using subpectoral carbon dioxide. Ann Thorac Surg 2006;81:1099—104.

36. Kobayashi S, Satoshi Y, Yuro K, et al. Correction of pectus excavatum and carinatum assisted by the endoscope. Plast Reconstr Surg 1997;99:1037—45.

37. Derveaux L, Clarysse T, Ivanoff T, et al. Preoperative and postoperative abnormalities in chest x-ray indices and in lung function in pectus deformities. Chest 1989;95:850—6.

38. Fonkalsrud EW. Management of pectus chest deformities in female patients. Am J Surg 2004;187:192—7.

39. Lester CW. Surgical treatment of protrusion deformities of the sternum and costal cartilages (pectus carinatum, pigeon breast). Ann Surg 1961;153:441—6.

40. Currarino G, Silverman N. Premature obliteration of the sternal sutures and pigeon breast deformity. Radiology 1958;70:532—40.

41. Chidambaram B, Mehta AV. Currarino-Silverman Syndrome (pectus carinatum Type 2 deformity) and mitral valve disease. Chest 1992;102:780—2.

42. Robicsek F. Marlex mesh support for the correction of very severe and recurrent pectus excavatum. Ann Thorac Surg 1978;26:80—3.

43. Nuss D, Kelly JR Jr, Croitoru DD, et al. A 10-year review of a minimally invasive technique for the correction of pectus excavatum. J Pediatr Surg 1998;33:545—52.

44. Abramson H, D'Agostino J, Wascovi S. A 5-year experience with a minimally invasive technique for pectus carinatum repair. J Pediatr Surg 2009;44:118—24.

45. Kim S, Idowu O. Minimally invasive thoracoscopic repair of unilateral pectus carinatum. J Pediatr Surg 2009;44:471—4.

46. Frey AS, Garcia VF, Brown RL, et al. Nonoperative management of pectus carinatum. J Pediatr Surg 2006;41:40—5.

47. Lee SY, Lee SJ, Jeon CW, et al. Effect of the compressive brace in pectus carinatum. Eur J Cardiothorac Surg 2008;34:146—9.

Thoracic Defects: Cleft Sternum and Poland Syndrome

Alexander A. Fokin, MD, PhD

KEYWORDS

• Chest wall defects • Cleft sternum • Poland syndrome

Defects of the thoracic cage with bone and/or muscle deficit are relatively rare. Besides the obvious cosmetic problems, they may also present a real risk depending on the severity of manifestations.

CLEFT STERNUM

Cleft sternum (CS), also known as sternum bifidum or sternal fissure, is a partial or complete failure of fusion of the sternal halves, which manifests itself as a midline defect of the sternum of different length and position.[1–3]

CS can be classified in main types (superior, subtotal, total, and inferior) and in rare types (median and CS with cleft mandible) (**Fig. 1**).[4] Most common are superior and subtotal CS (**Fig. 2**).

The condition is usually characterized by the defect in the upper part of the sternum that paradoxically deepens during inspiration and protrudes with expiration, cough, or Valsalva maneuver. The pulsating heart can be noticeable under the thin and sometimes ulcerated and infected skin. Craniofacial hemangiomas (more frequent in female patients) and supraumbilical midline raphe are common (**Fig. 3**).[5] Lung herniation at the upper part of the defect may occur during increases in intrathoracic pressure if intraclavicular diastasis (ranges from 2 to more than 6 cm) is wide (**Fig. 4**). An umbilical hernia or the diastasis of the rectus abdominis muscle may be present. The diagnosis is easily established postpartum. Prenatally, high-resolution ultrasonography may diagnose the condition and postnatally it helps to accurately evaluate cartilaginous parts of the sternum and possible cardiovascular malformations.[6] Intracardiac defects and aortic arch anomalies (aortic aneurysm, coarctation) are more common in cases of total CS where heart disease is reported with an incidence of 8%.[7] Intratracheal hemangioma and vascular lesions of the vertebrobasilar system should be excluded before surgery to avoid complications.[1,6,8] Inferior CS is often associated with pentalogy of Cantrell.[2]

Surgical treatment of CS is indicated for several reasons: (1) lack of bony protection makes the heart and great vessels susceptible to trauma; (2) ulceration of the thinned skin and possible dermopericardial connection may lead to infectious pericarditis; (3) paradoxic movements of the anterior chest wall may result in mediastinal displacement, right ventricular overload, arrhythmias, and so forth; (4) dyspnea, reduced lung aeration, and cough reflex could lead to more frequent respiratory infections; (5) the appearance of the protruding heart disturbs patients and parents; (6) possible enlargement of the defect over time makes its correction more difficult; and (7) umbilical hernia and rectus muscle diastasis requires correction that could be done simultaneously.[9]

Surgical correction is recommended during the neonatal period when a compliant thorax allows direct approximation of the sternal halves.[2,10,11] Simultaneous repair of cardiac malformations is also feasible.[12] During the course of the surgical procedure, the pericardium is separated from the skin. The perichondrium is carved of the sternal halves, turned inward, and sutured together, thus creating the posterior sternal lamina.[3] This technique also prepares the sternal edges for

Heineman Medical Research Foundation, 1001 Blythe Boulevard, Suite 604, Charlotte, NC 28203, USA
E-mail address: lisa.freeman@heineman.org

Thorac Surg Clin 20 (2010) 575–582
doi:10.1016/j.thorsurg.2010.06.001

CLASSIFICATION OF STERNAL CLEFTS
I. Main Types

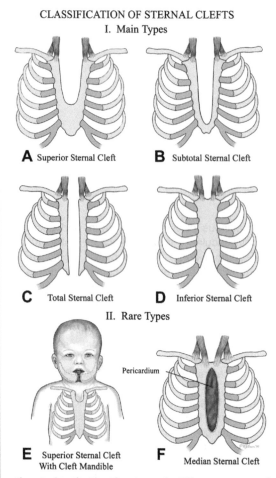

A Superior Sternal Cleft

B Subtotal Sternal Cleft

C Total Sternal Cleft

D Inferior Sternal Cleft

II. Rare Types

Pericardium

E Superior Sternal Cleft
With Cleft Mandible

F Median Sternal Cleft

Fig. 1. (*A–F*) Classification of different types of sternal clefts. Main types: (*A*) Superior sternal cleft. (*B*) Subtotal sternal cleft. (*C*) Total sternal cleft. (*D*) Inferior sternal cleft. Rare types: (*E*) Superior sternal cleft with cleft mandible. (F) Median sternal cleft. (*From* Fokin AA, Steuerwald NM, Ahrens WA, et al. Anatomic, histologic, and genetic characteristics of congenital chest wall deformities. Semin Thorac Cardiovasc Surg 2009;21(1):55.)

unification. Notching or wedging the sternal bars may ease their alignment before they are united using nonabsorbable interrupted sutures (**Figs. 5 and 6**).[13] In older patients and in cases of wider defects, the sliding chondrotomies are recommended to facilitate approximation and reduce the possibility of internal compression.[10] Wide cephaldal diastases may require mobilization of sternoclavicular junctions. In cases of subtotal CS, the distal cartilaginous bridge holding the halves apart should be resected. Although rarely needed, suturing of the muscles at the base of the neck may be implemented to prevent lung herniation.[3,14]

The first postoperative day is most crucial because of the possibility of compression caused by acute reduction of the mediastinal space.

When the defect is wide or in adult patients, the use of different patches (eg, Teflon, Gore-Tex, synthetic mesh, metal plate) or bone grafts has been successfully implemented.[2,15–17]

Sternal foramen (SF) is a localized and asymptomatic circular defect in the lower third of the sternum (more often singular but sometimes multiple) that is found in approximately 7% of the general population during CT or midline sternotomy. It occurs twice as often in male patients and is more prevalent in the black race.[18] Clinical implications require precautions to be used during sternal biopsy and acupuncture (needles fitted with guards) to prevent fatal damage to the right ventricle or aorta. In forensic medicine, SF can be used in skeletal identification and should not be mistaken for a gunshot wound or bone destruction caused by carcinoma or osteomyelitis.[19]

POLAND SYNDROME

Poland syndrome (PS) or pectoral aplasia–dysdactylia syndrome is one of the most intriguing and unique constellations of symptoms that combines unilateral defects of bones and muscles with possible internal organ malformations. PS is characterized by unilateral absence of the sternocostal head of the pectoralis major muscle, hypoplasia or absence of the pectoralis minor muscle, aplasia or hypoplasia of the costal cartilages of the second through the fifth ribs, hypoplasia or absence of the breast and nipple, alopecia of the axillary region, and ipsilateral brachysyndactyly (**Fig. 7**).[4] The degree and extent of the various components of the syndrome vary significantly and rarely does a single individual manifest all of its features. There is no correlation between the extent of the chest wall deformity and the hand malformations.[2,20]

This anomaly was first described in 1826 by L.M. Lallemand and then again in 1841 by Alfred Poland.[2] The estimated incidence of PS is 1 in 30,000 (with a range from 1 in 7000 to 1 in 100,000), depending on the severity of the condition and the patient population. In more common sporadic PS, there is a male prevalence (70%), as well as a right-side prevalence. In rare familial PS (approximately 30 cases described) there is no side or gender predominance.[21–23] PS is a nongenetic congenital abnormality with low risk of recurrence (<1%) in the same family.[24,25]

The pathogenesis of PS remains controversial. The descriptions of the reduced flow and hypoplasia of the corresponding vasculature support

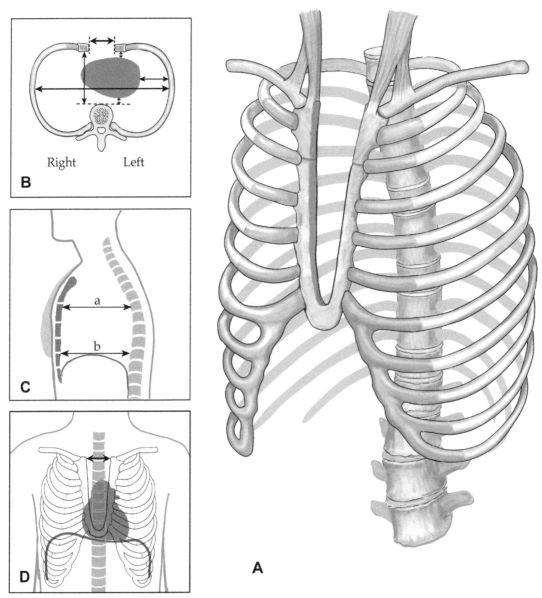

Fig. 2. (*A–D*) Anatomic representation of subtotal sternal cleft. (*A*) Three dimensional view. V-shaped sternal defect with distal cartilaginous bridge. (*B*) Cross-sectional view. Defect of the sternal bone with underlying heart. (*C*) Lateral view. Protrusion of the mediastinum. (*D*) Frontal view. V-shaped sternal defect with increased intraclavicular distance.

the prevailing theory of embryonic subclavian artery (SA) blood supply disruption, leading to the subsequent anatomic defects. Conversely, the reports of normal SA and internal thoracic arteries (ITA), confirmed by CT and flow measurements, imply that just transient flow interruptions during early organogenesis may trigger the malformations and that the disruption of a lateral plate mesoderm could be an underlying cause.[22,26–28]

PS can be classified into 3 groups: (1) mild or partial PS with only pectoralis muscle deficit (constitutive sign of the condition); (2) moderate or classic PS, which exhibits unilateral chest/hand deformity that includes pectoral muscle aplasia with chondro-costal hypoplasia and syndactyly; and (3) severe PS in which thoracic involvement broadens to include rib aplasia with lung herniation along with isolated dextrocardia

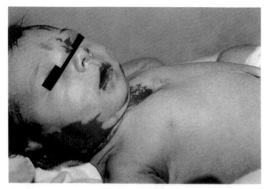

Fig. 3. Patient with superior sternal cleft, craniofacial hemangiomas, supraumbilical midline raphe, umbilical hernia. Paradoxic depression of the anterior chest wall at inspiration.

(in left-sided PS with rib agenesia), muscle deficit extends to include ipsilateral hypoplasia of the latissimus dorsi and deltoid muscles, ectrodactyly and sometimes ipsilateral renal agenesia, and so forth (**Fig. 8**).

Lung herniation occurs in approximately 8% of cases. Anteroposterior radiography usually demonstrates a unilateral hyperlucent lung. The flail anterior chest wall does not necessarily transform into the paradoxic mediastinal movements. Other rare causes of respiratory impairment in PS may include bullous emphysema, spontaneous pneumothorax, and congenital diaphragmatic hernia.[2,23]

Muscle deficit of the thoracic cage usually does not result in functional deficiency of the shoulder.[29]

Isolated dextrocardia (dextroposition without inversion) was documented in approximately 40 cases, all in left-sided PS with agenesia of more than 2 ribs (**Fig. 9**).[22,30]

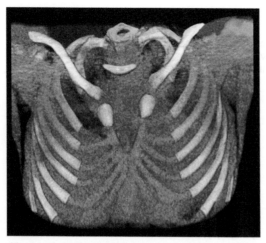

Fig. 4. CT image of superior cleft sternum. Wide V-shaped sternal defect.

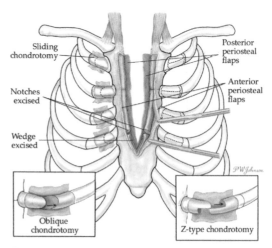

Fig. 5. Surgical correction of the superior sternal cleft. Formation of the perichondrial flaps for creation of posterior sternal lamina. Sliding chondrotomies. Notching of the sternal bars and midline wedge sternotomy for approximation of the sternal halves. (*From* Fokin AA, Robicsek F. Management of chest wall deformities. In: Franco KL, Putnam JB Jr, editors. Advanced therapy in thoracic surgery. 2nd edition. Shelton (CT): PMPH-USA, Ltd; 2005. p. 160; with permission.)

Hand involvement has been reported in 13.5% to 56.0% of patients and varies from mild shortness of the middle phalanges with cutaneous webbing to complete absence of the hand. Conversely, approximately 10% of patients with syndactyly have Poland's syndrome.[31,32]

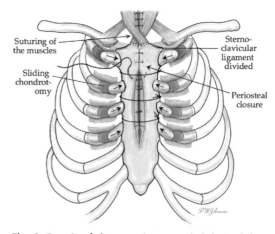

Fig. 6. Repair of the superior sternal cleft. Mobilization of the sternoclavicular junctions. Suturing of the perichondrial flaps. Crossing and suturing of the medial attachments of the sternocleidomastoid muscles. Union of the sternal halves. (*From* Fokin AA, Robicsek F. Management of chest wall deformities. In: Franco KL, Putnam JB Jr, editors. Advanced therapy in thoracic surgery. 2nd edition. Shelton (CT): PMPH-USA, Ltd; 2005. p. 160; with permission.)

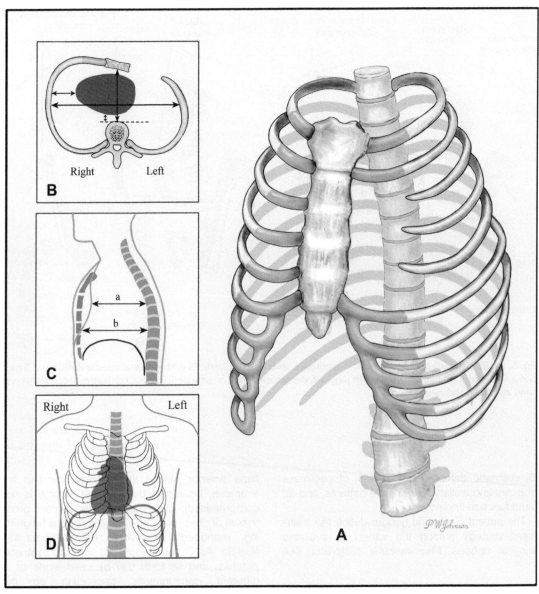

Fig. 7. (*A–D*) Anatomic representation of Poland syndrome. (*A*) Three-dimensional view. Left-sided rib defect. (*B*) Cross-sectional view. Rib defect with chest wall depression and shift of the heart to the right. (*C*) Lateral view. Unilateral chest wall depression. (*D*) Frontal view. Rib defect and isolated dextrocardia. (*From* Fokin AA, Steuerwald NM, Ahrens WA, et al. Anatomic, histologic, and genetic characteristics of congenital chest wall deformities. Semin Thorac Cardiovasc Surg 2009;21(1):55.)

There is a well-known association between PS and Mobius syndrome, Srengel's deformity, and Klippel-Feil syndrome.[25]

The relationship between PS and several malignancies has been documented to include an association with leukemia, non-Hodgkin's lymphoma, leiomyosarcoma, cervical cancer, neuroblastoma, Wilms tumor, and so forth. The hypoplasia of the breast does not exclude the development of invasive ductal carcinoma, thus requiring monitoring for early detection of cancer and appropriate treatment strategies.[2,33]

Surgical intervention is indicated for the following reasons: (1) asymmetric depression of the chest wall and the possibility of its enlargement, (2) lack of adequate protection for the heart and/or lungs, (3) paradoxic movement of the chest wall, (4) hypoplasia or aplasia of the female breast,

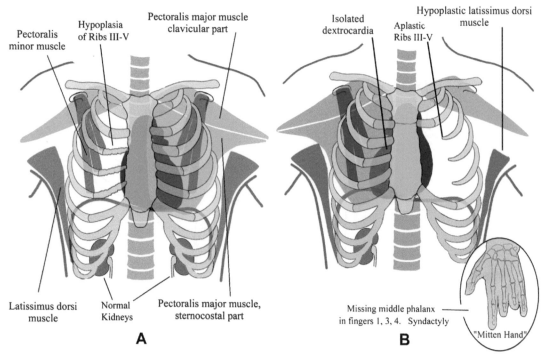

Pectoralis minor muscle

Hypoplasia of Ribs III-V

Pectoralis major muscle clavicular part

Isolated dextrocardia

Aplastic Ribs III-V

Hypoplastic latissimus dorsi muscle

Latissimus dorsi muscle

Normal Kidneys

Pectoralis major muscle, sternocostal part

Missing middle phalanx in fingers 1, 3, 4. Syndactyly

"Mitten Hand"

A　　　　　　　　　　B

Fig. 8. (*A*, *B*) Different degrees of Poland syndrome severity. (*A*) Classic PS with pectoral muscle deficit and hypoplasia of the ribs. (*B*) Full-blown PS with large rib defect, extensive muscle deficit, isolated dextrocardia, ipsilateral hand anomaly, and renal agenesia.

(5) cosmetic defect owing to lack of pectoralis muscles and axillary fold in male patients, and (6) hand function impairment.[13]

The patient's age and gender define the treatment strategy among the variety of available surgical options. Microvascular perforator free flaps (inferior gluteal artery perforator flap for example), latissimus dorsi flap (if muscle is not compromised), customized silicon breast prostheses or chest wall implants, autologous fat grafting, monopedic transverse rectus abdominis muscle flap, autologous rib grafts, synthetic patches, and so forth can be used alone or in different combinations depending on the case.[13,34–37] Each method has its own advantages/indications, limitations, and complications. The correction could be done in 1 (preferably) or 2 stages depending on the severity of the defect and the age of the patient.

A detailed assessment of ITA in patients with PS is mandatory, especially in planned coronary artery bypass graft surgery or muscle flap transplantation. The latter also requires MR or CT evaluation of the related muscle to exclude possible hypoplasia, even in the presence of normal appearance.[38]

Anesthetic management includes prevention of malignant hyperthermia, avoidance of succinylcholine and halothane, and implementation of positive pressure ventilation.[39] A double lumen endotracheal tube is recommended for unilateral

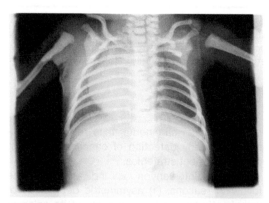

Fig. 9. Radiograph of the patient with left sided Poland's Syndrome, with the defect of 2 ribs and isolated dextrocardia. (*Courtesy of* Meir Mei-Zahav, MD, Israel.)

ventilation of the normal lung and to collapse the lung on the side of chest wall reconstruction for pulmonary injury prevention.[20]

REFERENCES

1. Eijgelaar A, Bijtel JH. Congenital cleft sternum. Thorax 1970;25:490–8.
2. Ravitch MM. Congenital deformities of the chest wall and their operative correction. Philadelphia: WB Saunders Company; 1977.
3. Bairov GA, Fokin AA. [The cleft sternum]. Vestn Khir Im Il Grek 1984;133(9):109–15 [in Russian].
4. Fokin AA, Steuerwald NM, Ahrens WA, et al. Anatomical, histologic, and genetic characteristics of congenital chest wall deformities. Semin Thorac Cardiovasc Surg 2009;21(1):44–57.
5. Gorlin RJ, Kantaputra P, Aughton DJ, et al. Marked female predilection in some syndromes associated with facial hemangiomas. Am J Med Genet 1994; 52(2):130–5.
6. Mazzie JP, Lepore J, Price AP, et al. Superior sternal cleft associated with PHACES syndrome: postnatal sonographic findings. J Ultrasound Med 2003; 22(3):315–9.
7. Shalak L, Kaddoura I, Obeid M, et al. Complete cleft sternum and congenital heart disease: review of the literature. Pediatr Int 2002;44(3):314–6.
8. Pascual-Castroviejo I. The association of extracranial and intracranial vascular malformations in children. Can J Neurol Sci 1985;12(2):139–48.
9. Fokin AA. Cleft sternum and sternal foramen. Chest Surg Clin N Am 2000;10(2):261–76.
10. Sabiston DC. The surgical management of congenital bifid sternum with partial ectopia cordis. J Thorac Surg 1958;35(1):118–22.
11. Jewett TC Jr, Butsch WL, Hug HR. Congenital bifid sternum. Surgery 1962;52(6):932–6.
12. Bové T, Goldstein JP, Viart P, et al. Combined repair of upper sternal cleft and tetralogy of Fallot in an infant. Ann Thorac Surg 1997;64(2):561–2.
13. Fokin AA, Robicsek F. Management of chest wall deformities. In: Franco KL, Putnam JB Jr, editors. Advanced therapy in thoracic surgery. 2nd edition. Hamilton (Canada): BC Decker; 2005. p. 145–62.
14. Daum R, Hecker WC. Operative correction of total sternum bifida. Thoraxchir Vask Chir 1964;12: 333–9.
15. Burton JF. Method of correction of ectopia cordis. Arch Surg 1947;54(1):79–84.
16. Hazari A, Mercer N, Pawade A, et al. Superior cleft sternum: construction with a titanium plate. Plast Reconstr Surg 1998;101(1):167–70.
17. Schmidt AI, Jesch NK, Gluer S, et al. Surgical repair of combined gastroschisis and sternal cleft. J Pediatr Surg 2005;40(6):e21–3.
18. McCormick WF. Sternal foramena in man. Am J Forensic Med Pathol 1981;2(3):249–52.
19. Schratter M, Bijak M, Nissel H, et al. Foramen sternale: minor anomaly—great significance. Fortschr Rontgenstr 1997;166(1):69–71.
20. Urchel HC Jr. Poland syndrome. Semin Thorac Cardiovasc Surg 2009;21(1):89–94.
21. Freire-Maia N, Chautard EA, Opitz JM, et al. The Poland syndrome: clinical and genealogical data, dermatoglyphic analysis, and incidence. Hum Hered 1973;23:97–104.
22. Bavinck JN, Weaver DD. Subclavian artery supply disruption sequence: hypothesis of a vascular etiology for Poland, Klippel-Feil, and Möbius anomalies. Am J Med Genet 1986;23(4):903–18.
23. Fokin AA, Robicsek F. Poland's Syndrome revisited. Ann Thorac Surg 2002;74(6):2218–25.
24. Stevens DB, Fink BA, Prevel C. Poland's syndrome in one identical twin. J Pediatr Orthop 2000;20(3):392–5.
25. Kuklik M. Poland-Mobius syndrome and disruption spectrum affecting the face and extremities: a review paper and presentation of five cases. Acta Chir Plast 2000;42(3):95–103.
26. Ailiwadi M, Arildsen RC, Greelish JP. Poland syndrome: a contraindication to the use of the internal thoracic artery in coronary artery bypass grafting? J Thorac Cardiovasc Surg 2005;130(2): 578–9.
27. Rosa RF, Travi GM, Valiatti F, et al. Poland syndrome associated with an aberrant subclavian artery and vascular abnormalities of the retina in a child exposed to misoprostol during pregnancy. Birth Defects Res A Clin Mol Teratol 2007;79:507–11.
28. Dustagheer S, Basheer MH, Collins A, et al. Further support for the vascular aetiology of Poland syndrome—a case report. J Plast Reconstr Aesthet Surg 2009;62(10):e360–1.
29. Bairov GA, Fokin AA. [Surgical treatment in Poland's syndrome in children]. Vestn Khir Im Il Grek 1994; 152(1–2):70–2 [in Russian].
30. Fraser FC, Teebi AS, Walsh S, et al. Poland sequence with dextrocardia: which comes first? Am J Med Genet 1997;73:194–6.
31. David TJ. Preaxial polydactyly and the poland complex [letter to the editor]. Am J Med Genet 1982; 13:333–4.
32. Al-Qattan MM. Classification of hand anomalies in Poland's syndrome. Br J Plast Surg 2001;54:132–6.
33. Katz SC, Hazen A, Colen SR, et al. Poland's syndrome and carcinoma of the breast: a case report. Breast J 2001;7(1):56–9.
34. Gautam AK, Allen RJ Jr, Lo Tempio MM, et al. Congenital breast deformity reconstruction using perforator flaps. Ann Plast Surg 2007;58(4):353–8.
35. Coleman SR, Saboeiro AP. Fat grafting to the breast revisited: safety and efficacy. Plast Reconstr Surg 2007;119(3):775–85.

36. Borschel GH, Constantino DA, Cederna PS. Individualized implant-based reconstruction of Poland syndrome breast and soft tissue deformities. Ann Plast Surg 2007;59(5):507–14.

37. Zhou F, Liu W, Tang Y. Autologous rib transplantation and terylene patch for repair of chest wall defect in a girl with Poland syndrome: a case report. J Pediatr Surg 2008;43(10):1902–5.

38. Cochran JH Jr, Pauly TJ, Edstrom LE, et al. Hypoplasia of the latissimus dorsi muscle complicating breast reconstruction in Poland's syndrome. Ann Plast Surg 1981;6(5):402–4.

39. Kabukcu HK, Sahin N, Kanevetci BN, et al. Anaesthetic management of patient with Poland syndrome and rheumatic mitral valve stenosis: a case report. Ann Card Anaesth 2005;8(2):145–7.

Indications and Technique of Nuss Procedure for Pectus Excavatum

Donald Nuss, MB, ChB, Robert E. Kelly Jr, MD*

KEYWORDS

- Pectus excavatum • Thoracoscopy • Nickel allergy
- Nuss procedure

Many modifications have been made to the minimally invasive pectus repair since it was first performed in 1987 and the 10-year experience published in the *Journal of Pediatric Surgery* in 1998.[1] The experience can be divided into the first decade with 42 patients treated at one institution and the second decade with several thousand patients treated worldwide at multiple institutions.[2–9] In the first decade, the modifications included changing the incision from an anterior chest incision to bilateral thoracic incisions and redesigning the pectus bar from a short, soft, square-ended strut to a much longer and stronger steel bar with rounded ends.[1]

In the second decade, many new features were added to make the procedure safer and more successful. These features included the routine use of thoracoscopy; the development of completely new instruments specifically designed for tunneling, bar rotation, and bar bending; the development of a stabilizer; and the placement of pericostal sutures around the bar and underlying ribs to prevent bar displacement.[9–12] The increase in the number of patients presenting for surgical correction was not only because of an increase in referral by primary care physicians but also because of self-referral by patients who obtained their information from the Internet.[12–14] This increase in numbers worldwide, combined with longer follow-up, allowed clarification of age limits, indications for surgery, and duration of bar placement.[6,8,9,12,14–19] In addition, complications have been more clearly defined and are divided into early and late groupings.[20–22] The effects of the early learning experience have been separated from those of the later experiences.[2,4,13,20–26] More studies comparing cardiopulmonary function[18,27–33] and quality of life[34–37] before and after surgery are now available. Long-term results after bar removal have confirmed that the excellent results achieved at the time of repair are maintained after bar removal.[7–9,11,12,38]

CLINICAL FEATURES

Pectus excavatum (PE) may be present at birth, but in the authors' series of more than 2000 patients, most presented during the pubertal growth spurt, of which 80% were boys (**Table 1**).[38] Associated scoliosis occurs in 20% to 30% of the patients,[38,39] and connective tissue disorders such as Marfan syndrome, Marfanoid features and Ehlers-Danlos syndrome occur in up to 20%.[38]

Morphology

The deformity most frequently involves the lower sternum and chest wall. Focal or cup-shaped depressions are the most common type; broad, shallow, saucer-shaped deformities are the second most frequent; a long furrow or trench, which is usually asymmetrical (Grand Canyon

Department of Surgery, Eastern Virginia Medical School, Children's Hospital of The King's Daughters, 601 Children's Lane, Suite 5B, Norfolk, VA 23507, USA
* Corresponding author.
E-mail address: Robert.Kelly@chkd.org

Thorac Surg Clin 20 (2010) 583–597
doi:10.1016/j.thorsurg.2010.07.002
1547-4127/10/$ — see front matter © 2010 Elsevier Inc. All rights reserved.

Table 1
Medical history of 327 patients studied

Condition	Number	Percentage
Exercise intolerance	211	64.5
Lack of endurance	205	62.7
Shortness of breath	203	62.1
Chest pain with exercise	167	51.1
Family history of PE	140	42.8
Chest pain without exercise	104	31.8
Asthma	70	21.4
Scoliosis	69	21.1
Cardiac abnormalities	65	19.9
Frequent or prolonged URI	44	13.5
Palpitations	37	11.3
Pneumonia	28	8.6
Fainting/dizziness	27	8.3
Marfan syndrome	15	4.6
Family history of PC	13	4.0
Ehlers-Danlos syndrome	9	2.8
Family history of Marfan syndrome	8	2.4
Patient adopted	4	1.2
Patient has identical twin	3	0.9
Family history of Ehlers-Danlos syndrome	2	0.6
Sprengel deformity	2	0.6

Abbreviations: PC, pectus carinatum; URI, upper respiratory infection.

From Kelly RE Jr. Pectus excavatum: historical background, clinical picture, preoperative evaluation and criteria for operation. Semin Pediatr Surg 2008; 17(3):210; with permission.

type), is the third most common; and mixed carinatum and excavatum deformities occur in 5%.[40]

Radiographic Evaluation

Because the morphology varies, preoperative imaging for anatomic assessment and documentation of dimensions of the chest are important. A routine chest radiograph is used in some centers[41] because it is inexpensive, readily available, and allows measurement of the indices of severity. The radiograph is also helpful in recurrent PE because it shows the extent of abnormal calcification of cartilages.

A computed tomographic (CT) scan of the chest without contrast gives a clearer picture of the deformity and the bony and cartilaginous skeleton in 3 dimensions and allows calculation of the CT index. The 3-dimensional reconstruction is useful in determining the number of bars that may be necessary, especially in diffuse deformities, which extend up toward the clavicles. Cartilaginous deformity is poorly seen on a chest radiograph but well visualized on a CT scan. Likewise, cardiac and pulmonary compressions as well as the relationship of the sternum to the compressed heart are much better visualized on the CT scan than on a chest radiograph. CT also helps better to see abnormal calcification of cartilages in a recurrent previous open (Ravitch) operation.[42] Review of the CT scan with the patient and parents before surgery helps to communicate the extent of deformity and to form expectations for the hospital course and final outcome. A method for measuring asymmetry and cephalad extension of the depression by CT scan has been published.[43]

Magnetic resonance imaging (MRI) may be used instead of CT to reduce radiation exposure, especially in children who are old enough to cooperate and do not require sedation or general anesthesia for MRI.

Daunt and colleagues[44] examined normal children to obtain values for the pectus index (2–2.3 in normal individuals). In 557 patients, it was found that the 0- to 2-year age group had a significantly smaller mean Haller (pectus) index than older children. In addition, girls had significantly greater pectus index values than boys in the 0- to 6-year and 12- to 18-year age groups. Following surgical correction, Kilda and colleagues[45] observed that the pectus index increased by 0.45 ± 0.49. Statistically significant index differences before and after surgery were not detected in 88 children when the preoperation pectus index was less than 3.12 ($P = .098$). The investigators recommended indications for surgical treatment based on improvement in values for several radiographic indices after operation. Kilda and colleagues state that the commonly used pectus index should be greater than 3.1.

Exercise Limitation

Many patients with PE have a perceived limitation of exercise ability.[30,37] Investigations of exercise ability have yielded mixed results. Over more than 50 years, there have been dozens of studies of cardiac or pulmonary function in PE. In 2006, Malek and associates[30] reported a meta-analysis based on a computer-assisted search of the literature. The investigators concluded that surgical repair improved cardiovascular function. Sigalet and colleagues[32] studied patients pre-and postrepair and reported significant improvement in cardiac stroke volume, cardiac output, forced expiratory volume in the first second of expiration (FEV_1), total lung capacity (TLC), TLC (percentage expected), diffusing lung capacity, maximum oxygen consumption (Vo_2max), respiratory quotient, and O_2 pulse (percentage predicted).

Pulmonary Function Studies

Efforts to elicit the cause of exercise intolerance have led to studies of pulmonary function at rest, including spirometry and plethysmography. Results of spirometry in patients with PE are usually 10% to 20% less than the expected average for the population. Plethysmography shows that lung volumes are similarly decreased (**Fig. 1**).[46–48] At the authors' institution, in 855 patients with PE presenting for surgical treatment, the mean forced vital capacity (FVC) was only 77% instead of the 100% predicted value, the mean FEV_1 was 83%, and the forced expiratory flow, midexpiratory phase ($FEF_{25\%-75\%}$) was 73%. In the same group, 26% of the patients had an FVC in the abnormal category, less than the 80% predicted value, and for FEV_1 and $FEF_{25\%-75\%}$, the number in the abnormal range was even higher, with 32% and 45%, respectively, whereas in the normal distribution, only 16% of the patients should have less than the 80% predicted value ($P<.001$). In 327 patients enrolled in a multicenter study of PE, FVC for patients aged 8 to 21 years was a mean 90% of the predicted value; FEV_1, 89%; and $FEF_{25\%-75\%}$, 85%. These decreases are statistically and clinically significant ($P<.001$) (see Fig. 1).[12,28,33] In a study of patients with recurrent PE, the predicted values showed significant restrictive disease in more than half of the patients.[49]

Cardiology Evaluation

Cardiological evaluation is important because a significant number of patients have findings of right atrial and ventricular compression, mitral valve prolapse, and rhythm abnormalities. Also, because many patients with PE have exercise-related symptoms, including chest pain, it is useful to assure normal heart functioning when planning a major thoracic operation. Mitral valve prolapse was present in 17% of the patients in the authors' series and in up to 65% of those in other series, as opposed to only 1% in the normal pediatric population.[50–52] Mitral valve prolapse as a direct consequence of compression is suggested by CT scan[53] and confirmed by its resolution in half of the surgically treated cases. Dysrhythmias, including first-degree heart block, right bundle branch block, or Wolff-Parkinson-White syndrome, were present in 16% of the authors' patients.[54]

The hemodynamic effects of PE have been the subject of numerous reports and much controversy. The amount of right atrial and ventricular compressions varies with the overall shape of the chest.[55] These effects were reported first several years ago, but more recent imaging and exercise/work/oxygen uptake techniques are clarifying previous findings. Using angiography, Garusi and D'Ettorre[56] demonstrated displacement of the heart to the left side with a sternal imprint on the anterior wall of the right ventricle.[50,56] This finding is now easily verified noninvasively by CT or MRI.

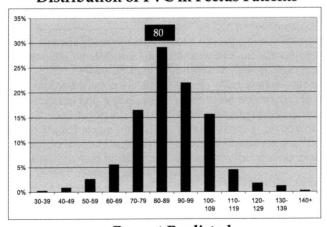

Distribution of FVC in Pectus Patients

Percent Predicted

Fig. 1. Preoperative resting pulmonary function studies in 900 patients with PE showing the peak for FVC shifted to the left. The graph should peak at 100% of predicted value and not at 80%. (*From* Nuss D. Minimally invasive surgical repair of pectus excavatum. Semin Pediatr Surg 2008;17(3):215; with permission.)

In 1962, Bevegard[57] found that work capacity was related to the severity of the pectus depression. Evaluating 16 patients via right heart catheterization, he found that patients with a 20% or greater decrease in physical work capacity had a shorter distance from the sternum to the vertebrae. The decrease in stroke volume on changing from a supine to sitting posture at rest was similar to that of normal subjects (40%). The increase in stroke volume from rest to exercise was only 18.5%, much less than the 51% increase in normal subjects (P<.001). Thus a measured lower work capacity was found at any given heart rate while sitting.[50,57] Beseir and colleagues[58] performed cardiac catheterization on 6 patients and showed that stroke volume was 31% lower and cardiac output was 28% lower during upright and supine exercises. Postoperation, 3 patients had a 38% increase in the cardiac index, entirely because of an increase in stroke volume.[58]

The effect of mechanical compression by the sternum on the heart was demonstrated by Heitzer and Wollschlager[59] in a patient with a severe deformity and ischemic changes correlated by catheterization, CT scan, and electrocardiogram (ECG).[58] The occurrence of cor pulmonale and chronic respiratory acidosis is rare, but these conditions have been reported in a patient with PE in whom no other cause was uncovered after an extensive diagnostic workup.[60]

The narrower the chest in anteroposterior direction the more the heart is apt to be squeezed between the sternum and spine and the stroke volume diminished, as has been demonstrated by direct cardiac catheterization, oxygen saturation studies, CT scanning, and echocardiogram.[30,32,61] Improvement after operation has been demonstrated.[30,32,61] One of the reasons for persisting controversy concerning cardiac effects of PE until recently is the failure to objectively measure the severity of the chest depression and correlate it to the amount of cardiac compression. Kinuya and colleagues,[29] Sigalet and colleagues,[32] Coln and colleagues[31] and other researchers have clearly demonstrated the relief of cardiac compression.

In summary, compression of the right side of the heart, leading to a diminished stroke volume, combined with a modest lung restriction, leads to a diminished cardiopulmonary capacity in severe cases.

Body Image

Concern about the appearance of the chest prompts many patients to seek repair. A large percentage of patients with PE are extremely self-conscious about their chests; these patients withdraw from social and sports activities and become depressed and even suicidal. Children and adolescents with visible physical differences are at risk for developing body image issues and interpersonal difficulties because they are teased by their peers, which further aggravates the problem.[62] Nevertheless, patients with PE are often dismissed by pediatricians as having an inconsequential problem.[35,63] Pediatricians frequently tell children and parents that the chest wall deformity is only cosmetic and will resolve spontaneously. For this reason, the authors have sought to quantify psychosocial functioning with psychometrically sound assessments and to detect the effects of surgical correction of PE by this method. In collaboration with a psychologist with expertise in body image issues, a test for body image effects specific to PE was developed and validated.[34,37] Other researchers subsequently used this or similar psychometric testing tools and corroborated the findings.[15,64] Using the carefully developed and administered instrument, the multicenter study of PE evaluated more than 300 children younger than 21 years before and after operation. Marked improvement in psychosocial functioning was identified postrepair.[37] Several investigators have reported that the severity of the depression as measured by CT scan did not correlate with the patient's or parent's perception of body image concerns, which confirmed previous work on this topic.[65–67]

PREOPERATIVE CONSIDERATIONS

After confirming that the patient's condition is severe enough to fulfill the criteria for surgical correction as outlined earlier, several other factors need to be considered (Box 1; Fig. 2).

Age

The minimally invasive repair has been performed successfully on patients from age 1 year to older than 50 years.[6,8,10,12,14–19] The ideal age is just before puberty because at that age the chest is still malleable, the support bar is in place during the pubertal growth spurt, the recovery time is short, and the incidence of recurrence is low.[9,20] Patients younger than 8 years also have an excellent result and short recovery time, but because the support bar is removed before the pubertal growth spurt, there is a potential for recurrence.[9,12,38] However, if a young patient has significant cardiac and/or pulmonary compression, an early repair is justified, but the bar should be left in situ for 3 years. The family needs to be informed that the patient may require a second bar placement either at the time of removal of the first bar, when a longer bar may be inserted by using a chest tube switch technique or later if the condition recurs. Recurrence rate is less than 5% (**Table 2**). During the first decade, the minimally invasive procedure was used only in prepubertal patients, but experience has shown that postpubertal patients tolerate the procedure well; excellent results have been reported in patients in their 30s and 40s.[9,12,15–19] The older patients require 2 or more bars in more than 50% of the cases.[9,12]

Phenotype

The ideal chest configurations for the minimally invasive repair are the diffuse saucer shape, localized cup shape, and symmetric funnel shape.[9] Patients who have very steep cup-shaped depressions and those with severe deep, asymmetric, Grand Canyon–type depressions are more of a challenge and often require 2 bars. Park and colleagues[6] and other researchers[7] have suggested using an asymmetric bar in these patients. In patients in whom the depression mostly involves the upper chest, care needs to be taken not to place the bar too high because such placement will interfere with the axilla and its vital structures. Patients who have mixed excavatum and carinatum deformities may have residual protrusion of the carinatum after bar placement, especially if there is severe sternal torsion. Older patients have a higher incidence of sternal torsion and mixed deformities, which may be a good reason to perform the repair before puberty.[17,67,68] Patients who have Currarino-Silverman syndrome or pouter pigeon deformity with anterior displacement of the manubrium and posterior displacement of the gladiolus develop increased protrusion of the manubrium when the gladiolus is elevated with a substernal bar. Therefore, the minimally invasive procedure is not recommended in this category of patients.

Preoperative Preparation

If the patient has a history of nickel allergy, which occurs in 2% of the population, a titanium bar should be used.[69] The titanium bar needs to be ordered from the manufacturer before surgery (Biomet Microfixation, Jacksonville, FL, USA).

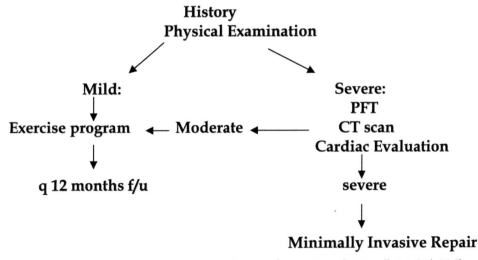

Clinical Algorithm

History
Physical Examination

Mild:

Exercise program ← Moderate ← Severe:
PFT
CT scan
Cardiac Evaluation

q 12 months f/u   severe

Minimally Invasive Repair

Fig. 2. Indications for PE repair. f/u, follow-up; PFT, pulmonary function test. (*From* Kelly RE, Cash TF, Shamberger RC, et al. Surgical repair of pectus excavatum markedly improves body image and perceived ability for physical activity: multicenters study. Pediatrics 2008;122:1218–22; with permission.)

Table 2
Long-term results after bar removal

Overall Results for Primary Repairs	
Total number of primary repairs	1235
Total number with bar removed	903
Excellent result	773 (85.6%)
Good result	99 (11.0%)
Fair result	11 (1.2%)
Poor result	6 (0.7%)
Failed	11 (1.2%)
Bar removed elsewhere	3 (0.3%)

Data collected through December 18, 2009.

The manufacturer needs to know the length of the bar required, and a copy of the CT scan at the insertion site is required so that the bar can be prebent.

All the usual precautions for insertion of a foreign body into a patient need to be meticulously adhered to. Pain management is discussed with the patient and family preoperatively.

POSITIONING THE PATIENT

The standard position is supine with both arms abducted at the shoulders to approximately 70°, taking care to protect the patient from brachial plexus injury. An alternative method includes elevating the torso on a mattress and extending the arms posteriorly.[22,70] This position allows insertion of the thoracoscope superior to the incision site but has the disadvantage of overextending the chest during the surgery. Another alternative position is to flex the left shoulder and elbow anteriorly, adjacent to the head,[71] but there have been anecdotal reports of brachial plexus injury with this position.

THORACOSCOPY

Thoracoscopy has become a routine part of the minimally invasive procedure.[11,12,23,71–73] Most surgeons use right-sided thoracoscopy,[12,23] others prefer left-sided thoracoscopy,[71] some use bilateral thoracoscopy,[74,75] and some insert the scope and introducer through the same thoracostomy sites.[76] In patients with extremely deep depressions, it may be necessary to use bilateral thoracoscopy because the heart is not only compressed but also displaced to the left, which impedes visibility from the right. Insertion of the trocar from the left when the heart is displaced in

that direction requires great caution. The trocar is usually inserted inferior to the incision sites, but it can be inserted through the incision site[13,71] or even superior to the incision site when the arm is extended posteriorly.[22,40] The trocar insertion site affects visibility, and the inferior insertion site allows for good visibility not only during the tunneling but also for suture placement during bar stabilization. The authors use blunt instrumentation for trocar insertion and direct the trocar in a superior direction to avoid the liver and diaphragm.[23]

The introducer tip should always be kept in view through the thoracoscope during mediastinal tunneling. If the tip cannot be visualized because the depression is too deep, the scope may be inserted from the opposite side or a more superior tunnel should be first created where the depression is not so deep. A 30° or flexible scope is helpful in this situation.

The carbon dioxide (CO_2) insufflation pressure should be kept as low as possible, and usually, a pressure of 5 mm Hg is sufficient to keep the lungs out of the operative field. When 2 bars are being inserted, there is more leakage, requiring a higher flow rate to keep the pressure up.

SKIN INCISION SITE

During the early days of the procedure, the anterior thoracic incision used for open repairs was also used for the minimally invasive procedure. However, this incision resulted in keloid formation because of tension on the wound, and it was difficult to place the bar ends into the subcutaneous pouch without extending it all the way across the chest. It was therefore decided to insert the bar through 2 small lateral thoracic incisions.[1] Transverse lateral thoracic incisions have the advantage of providing good access to the thoracostomy entry and exit sites, run parallel to the lines of tension (Langer lines), rarely cause keloid formation, and require minimal subcutaneous dissection. Vertical incisions in the mid or posterior axillary lines give poor access to the anterior chest wall and tend to cause keloid formation. When placing 2 or more bars, making a separate incision for each bar facilitates bar stabilization and bar removal after 3 years. In mature female patients, the incisions should be placed in the inframammary crease between the 6- and 9-o'clock positions and extended laterally if necessary. The inframammary incisions give excellent access to the anterior chest wall, even allowing insertion of 2 bars, and give an excellent cosmetic result because the incisions virtually disappear.

TUNNELING

The thoracic entry and exit sites should be placed close to the sternum to prevent disruption of the intercostal muscles. Ideally, the tunnel should pass right under the deepest point of the depression. If the deepest point of the deformity is inferior to the body of the sternum, the patient requires 2 bars: one under the sternum and the other under the deepest point of the depression. The introducer tip should always be kept in view during the tunneling. If the depression is too deep to keep the introducer at such a position, the first tunnel should be created more superiorly, leaving the introducer in place to elevate the sternum. Alternatively, the sternum can be elevated by using the suction cup[77] or by lifting it with a towel clamp or heavy suture.

An extrapleural approach has been advocated by Schaarschmidt and colleagues[74] to prevent pleural and pericardial reaction, with good preliminary results. This approach is technically more difficult, and the internal mammary vessels are at increased risk of being injured.

STERNAL ELEVATION

When the introducer is in position across the mediastinum, it is lifted in an anterior direction to pull the sternum and anterior chest wall out of their depressed position, thereby correcting the PE. Repeating this lifting maneuver numerous times loosens up the anterior chest wall, prevents substernal trauma, intercostal muscle injury caused by bar rotation, and minimizes the pressure on the bar, which decreases the risk of bar displacement and postoperative discomfort. The PE should be completely corrected before removing the introducer.

BAR STABILIZATION

Bar stabilization is essential for a successful outcome. When the minimally invasive technique was first developed, bar stabilization was attempted by creating a muscular pocket.[1] This technique resulted in a 15% bar displacement rate. Subsequently, a stabilizer or footplate was developed and attached to the bar to give it more stability.[11] Initially, the stabilizer was held in position only with fascial sutures, but it frequently became detached from the bar, so a wire suture was used to lash the stabilizer to the bar. Recently, the wire has been replaced with a braided polyblend suture called the FiberWire (Arthrex Inc, Naples, FL, USA), which is soft and much easier to apply than the wire. However, even with a stabilizer attached, the bar is dislodged in some

patients during the first 3 weeks before scar tissue can be laid down, and therefore additional support is needed during those first few weeks after surgery. Hebra and colleagues[10] were the first to advocate placing a suture around the bar and underlying ribs and called it the "third point fixation." The investigators advocated placing the suture adjacent to the sternum through a small stab wound. Most surgeons now use the lateral thoracic incision to place sutures around the bar and rib under thoracoscopic control.[8,9,78] Some centers use wire instead of absorbable sutures,[6,25,69,74] which increases the risk of injury to the underlying lung, especially if the wire fractures.[68]

NUMBER OF BARS

Initially, the procedure was done only on young patients, so only 1 bar was necessary.[1] However, now that the procedure is being used more commonly in postpubertal patients, numerous investigators have reported that 2 bars give better and more stable results.[1,8,9,12] Patients with Marfan syndrome, asymmetric Grand Canyon–type deformities, and wide saucer-shaped deformities; older or postpubertal patients; and patients in whom the procedure needs to be repeated also usually require 2 bars.[1,7,9,12,67] A second bar should be inserted if the repair is suboptimal after insertion of 1 bar. On the operating table, the correction always looks better than it does when the patient resumes normal posture because the normal thoracic lordosis is eliminated on the operating table. The authors have never regretted placing a second bar but have often regretted placing only one.

BAR AND CHEST CONFIGURATION

Many patients require a reoperation because the condition was initially undercorrected. It is important to slightly overcorrect the deformity to prevent buckling of the anterior chest wall and to decrease the risk of recurrence. The bar should therefore be semicircular with only a 2- to 4-cm flat section in the middle to support the sternum. The thoracostomy entry and exit sites into and out of the chest should be medial to the top of the pectus ridge on each side. A bar that is bent only at each end (table top configuration) gives insufficient correction and may allow the lung to herniate between the bar and anterior chest wall. The bar should not be too tight on the sides of the chest because it will cause painful rib and muscle erosion and the patient will outgrow the bar too soon, necessitating early bar removal.[7,26] In patients with asymmetric deformities, Park and colleagues[6] have recommended using an asymmetric bar, which gives more lift on the side of the asymmetric deformity.[8]

REOPERATION

Reoperations on failed previous repairs have been successfully accomplished in 51 previous Nuss repairs, 39 previous Ravitch repairs, 4 failed Ravitch and Nuss repairs, and 3 previous Leonard repairs. Thoracoscopy is particularly important in these groups of patients because they usually require lysis of adhesions before the tunneling can commence, which requires additional port placement.[75,79] A postoperative chest tube is helpful in managing the inevitable lung leak and oozing that follows the lysis of pulmonary adhesions. The failed Ravitch procedures may be classified into 2 categories, those in which there was a simple cave-in after the open repair, which is easily corrected with a substernal bar, and those in which there is diffuse osteochondrodystrophy, a condition that is not amenable to correction with a substernal bar because of excessive calcification and rigidity of the chest wall. In this group of patients in whom the Ravitch procedure failed and there was severe recurrence, acquired asphyxiating chondrodystrophy, and a rigid chest wall, there were 2 cases of temporary arrhythmic arrests that were thought to be caused by pressure of the introducer on the heart. Both patients were resuscitated, but in one patient sternotomy was required because the rigid calcified chest wall did not allow external cardiac compression. Complications are higher in the group of patients requiring reoperation: 55% required chest tubes, 8% had hemothorax, 8% had pleural effusion requiring drainage, and 2 had temporary arrhythmic arrest as mentioned earlier. The results were excellent in 66%, good in 30%, and fair in 2%, and the procedure failed in 2%, which is less satisfactory than the primary repair group.[3,67,79]

Prior thoracic surgery and concomitant open or thoracoscopic intrathoracic procedures have been successfully performed in conjunction with the minimally invasive PE repair.[80]

PAIN MANAGEMENT

A preemptive pain management protocol is used to prevent the pain cascade from being triggered. All patients receive lorazepam on the night before the surgery so that they will arrive at the hospital well rested and less anxious. In the presurgical holding area, midazolam is administered orally 45 minutes before the patient is taken to the operating room. After induction of anesthesia, a dose of intravenous ketorolac is given, and this drug is continued every 6 hours until day 3. While the patient is receiving the ketorolac, the intravenous fluids are kept at maintenance level to flush the kidneys and famotidine is given to prevent gastritis and gastrointestinal ulceration. In addition, blood urea and creatinine levels are checked on postoperative days 1 and 3. Until recently, an epidural infusion of fentanyl and bupivacaine was used, which was started during induction of anesthesia and continued until postoperative day 3 or 4. However, because 2 of 1300 patients developed partial paralysis, patient-controlled analgesia pumps are now used postoperatively. Patients also receive low-dose diazepam for muscle relaxation and anxiolysis. Stool softeners and laxatives are used prophylactically starting on day 1 to prevent constipation. Patients are discharged on day 4 or 5, with oxycodone and ibuprofen for pain control and diazepam and Robaxin for muscle relaxation.

Patients may return to school whenever they are strong enough; the duration varies with age, because prepubertal children recover quicker and are usually ready to return to school in 2 weeks, whereas postpubertal patients require 3 weeks. All patients are restricted from participating in sporting activities for 6 weeks, at which time they may recommence aerobic activities, and competitive sports may be resumed at 12 weeks postrepair.

EARLY POSTOPERATIVE COMPLICATIONS

Early complications (**Table 3**) have been markedly reduced by meticulous attention to fitness for surgery, surgical technique, bar stabilization, evacuation of the pneumothorax, incentive spirometry, and prophylactic antibiotics. Many centers have reported marked improvement in the complication rate after the early learning experience.[11,13,20,21,24]

An insignificant apical pneumothorax secondary to CO_2 insufflation for thoracoscopy is usually present on the initial chest radiograph and resolves spontaneously. A chest tube was inserted in 3% of the patients, usually because the CO_2 was not adequately removed or because there was a leak in the system before removal of the trocar and the surgeon elected to leave a chest tube rather than take the risk of having to insert one later. These pneumothoraxes resolve spontaneously and are really a part of the operation rather than true complications because there is no lung leak in a primary pectus repair. However, redo operations with lysis of pulmonary adhesions frequently do require a postoperative chest tube

Table 3
Early postoperative complications of patients undergoing primary surgery

Complication	% (Number of Patients)
Pneumothorax with spontaneous resolution	66.0 (746)
Pneumothorax with chest tube	4.4 (50)
Horner syndrome with spontaneous resolution	15.2 (188)
Drug reaction	3.2 (39)
Suture site infection	0.9 (11)
Pneumonia	0.7 (8)
Hemothorax	0.5 (6)
Pericarditis	0.5 (5)
Pleural effusion (requiring drainage)	0.3 (4)
Temporary paralysis	0.1 (1)
Cardiac perforation	—
Death	—

Data collected through December 18, 2009.

because these patients do have an air leak.[75,79] Pneumonia is rare in these young patients (0.5%), but postoperative incentive spirometry is vigorously encouraged, and all patients are given prophylactic antibiotics (cefazolin) for 24 hours. Wound and/or bar infection can be prevented if all the precautions for foreign body insertion are meticulously adhered to, and such infections have occurred in less than 1% of patients.[81-83] Infection requires vigorous treatment consisting of wound drainage, cultures, and appropriate intravenous antibiotics, followed by long-term oral antibiotics (sulfamethoxazole/trimethoprim). Treatment is usually effective in saving the bar if it is continued until the erythrocyte sedimentation rate (ESR) and C-reactive protein (CRP) level have returned to normal.[81-83] There have been reports of an increased infection rate on the side with the stabilizer,[84] but that has not been encountered by the authors in more than a thousand cases.

Pericarditis has occurred in 0.5% of the patients.[69,85,86] The cause is unclear. The condition appears to be caused by nickel allergy because it has not been seen in more than 6 years when screening patients more closely for nickel allergy was started. These patients present with persistent central chest pain, malaise, lethargy, and a pericardial friction rub. If an echocardiogram confirms the presence of pericardial fluid, the patient should be treated with a short course of prednisone. A pleural effusion that lasts for more than 4 days may also be caused by nickel allergy and should be treated similarly after aspirating fluid for culture. If symptoms recur after prednisone has been discontinued, the patient should be tested for nickel allergy (T.R.U.E Test by Allerderm Laboratories, Inc, Phoenix, AZ, USA). If the result is positive, low-dose prednisone can be given on alternate days until the ESR and CRP return to normal levels; if this option is unsuccessful, the steel bar is replaced with a titanium bar, which has only been necessary in 2 patients out of 1123 repairs.

Cardiac perforation has occurred in several centers during the early learning experience and before thoracoscopy was widely available.[6,87-90] Reviewing the preoperative CT scan to determine the position of the heart and its relationship to the sternum is helpful in planning the procedure, especially in patients with severe asymmetry and sternal torsion. If it appears that the heart is severely compressed, elevating the sternum with a hook or suction cup during the tunneling greatly minimizes the risk of injury. In addition, first tunneling 1 or 2 intercostal spaces superior to the deepest point and leaving the introducer in place to keep the sternum elevated while creating the second tunnel also minimizes the risk of pericardial or cardiac injury. The tip of the introducer should always be kept in sight. Good visibility with the thoracoscope in place is essential, and if necessary, bilateral thoracoscopy should be used.

It should be noted that with a substernal bar in place, cardioversion requires placement of the paddles in an anteroposterior position so that the current will be conducted through the heart. If the paddles are placed anterior and lateral then the current will simply be conducted along the bar and not through the heart.[88]

LATE COMPLICATIONS

Bar displacement has been the biggest late challenge. The initial bar displacement rate was 18.5% (**Table 4**). After the introduction of stabilizers, the rate dropped to 7.4%, and with the addition of pericostal sutures placed around the bar and underlying ribs, the rate dropped to 2%, only half of whom required revision (**Fig. 3**).[9,12,20]

The standard procedure is to place a stabilizer attached to the bar, with FiberWire suture on the left and multiple double-stranded "0" polydioxanone pericostal (PDS) sutures around the bar and underlying ribs on the right. If feasible, pericostal sutures are also placed on the left. If displacement is less than 20°, it can be observed by obtaining

Table 4
Late postoperative complications of patients who had primary surgery

Complication	Number of Patients	Percentage
Bar displacements	70	5.7
Requiring revision	50	4.1
Overcorrection	42	3.4
Bar allergy	38	3.1
Wound infection	18	15
Recurrence	13	1.1
Hemothorax	2	0.2
Skin erosion	1	0.1
Accidental death[a]	1	0.1

Data collected through December 18, 2009.
  Total number of patients, 1235.
  [a] Accidental death occurred after 3.5 years.

another chest radiograph in 1 month, and if there is no further progression, surgical revision is not usually required; however, if the displacement is more than 20° or it occurs right after surgery, it needs correction. At present, less than 1% of the patients require revision because of bar displacement.

Nickel allergy, which is present in 2%[69,85] of the population, may manifest early with pericarditis or persistent pleural effusion or may occur late with erythema of the anterior chest wall or inflammation and drainage at the incision sites. The inflammation and drainage may resemble a chronic infection, but cultures give a negative result and testing for nickel allergy gives a positive result. Treatment consists of local wound care and a short trial of prednisone. If the patient responds, administration of low-dose alternate-day prednisone until the ESR and CRP are back to normal levels usually resolves the problem. If the patient responds to the steroid therapy, the bar is left in place until it is time for removal. If the patient does not respond to treatment, the steel bar needs to be replaced with a titanium bar.[69,85] In the series of 1123 patients, 35 patients (3.1%) had allergy, of whom 22 were diagnosed preoperatively and received a titanium bar. Of the 13 who had a steel bar inserted, 10 were treated successfully with prednisone and 3 required bar removal.

Overcorrection, resulting in pectus carinatum, has occurred in 0.4% of the patients. These patients had Marfan syndrome and very deep cup-shaped deformities. Early bar removal was successful in 1 patient, and 2 required an external pressure brace. Other researchers have reported on carinatum developing especially in patients with asymmetry and a twisted sternum.[25]

Undercorrection not only predisposes the patients to increased risk of recurrence but also results in abnormal ridges developing adjacent to the sternum because there is not enough space. The cartilaginous portion of the rib will buckle under the pressure.

Persistent pain may be caused by bar displacement, stabilizer dislocation, bar being too tight or too long, sternal or rib erosion, infection, or allergy. An anterior and lateral chest radiograph, complete blood cell count, ESR, CRP level, and T.R.U.E. Test for allergy will identify the cause and allow appropriate treatment.

One accidental death occurred 3.5 years after pectus repair and was unrelated to the pectus surgery because the patient fell off an eighth-story balcony during a graduation celebration.

RESULTS

Long-term results 1 year after bar removal in the 903 patients who underwent primary repair are excellent in 773 patients (85.6%), good in 99 (11.0%), fair in 11 (1.2%), and poor in 6 (0.7%); the procedure failed in 11 patients (1.2%) and bar removal was done elsewhere in 3 patients

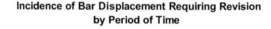

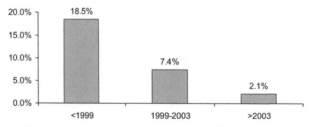

Fig. 3. Improvement in bar displacement rate over time as new modifications were introduced.

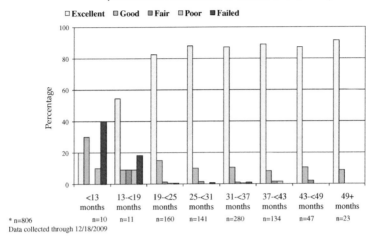

**Long-Term Results
by Length of Time Bar in Situ
(Bar Removed before December 31, 2008)**

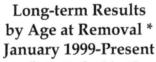

Fig. 4. Long-term results show that the bar should remain in situ for 2 to 4 years. The longer the bar remains in place the lower the recurrence rate up to 4 years.

(0.3%). (see **Table 2; Figs. 4** and **5**). Similar results have been reported by other centers.[5–8]

If the bar is removed before 2 years, the recurrence rate increases inversely with the length of time the bar remains in situ (see **Fig. 4**).

The age at the time of repair affects the recurrence rate. If the repair is performed in the very young, aged 5 years or younger, there is an increased risk of recurrence, although age is not as important as the duration of bar placement and should not prevent repair in a young patient with a severe PE with cardiac or pulmonary compression (see **Figs. 4** and **5**).[9] The higher recurrence rate in children aged 5 years and younger is mostly because these patients underwent repair during the learning curve, when patients did not keep their bars in place for the now standard 2 to 4 years.

All patients are encouraged to exercise regularly starting 6 to 8 weeks postoperatively. It is thought that patients who exercise regularly are more likely to maintain their excellent result than patients who are sedentary and rarely expand their chest to full capacity.

Postoperative cardiopulmonary function has been shown to have good improvement in some

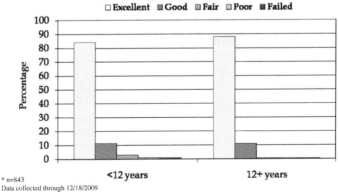

**Long-term Results
by Age at Removal ***
January 1999-Present

Fig. 5. Graph showing slightly improved results in older patients.

Distribution of FVC (After Bar Removal)

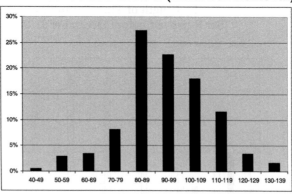

Percent Predicted

Fig. 6. Postoperative resting pulmonary function studies showing that the peak for FVC has shifted toward normal. (*From* Nuss D. Minimally invasive surgical repair of pectus excavatum. Semin Pediatr Surg 2008;17 (3):215; with permission.)

studies and less so in others. Several studies have shown significant improvement in pulmonary function postoperatively,[27–29,31–33,40] whereas others have shown no significant change.[19] The reasons for this discrepancy are multifactorial and include the size of the cohort being studied, the duration of the study, the severity of the PE, and whether the studies were done during exercise or at rest. In the authors' series of more than 900 cases, the preoperative resting pulmonary studies showed a marked shift to the left and a significant correction postoperatively (see **Fig. 1**; **Fig. 6**)[26,31]:

Postoperative cardiac studies have shown an increase in cardiac filling and stroke volume.[30–33] There is a discrepancy between the overwhelming number of patients reporting dramatic improvement in their exercise tolerance and the results of cardiac and pulmonary studies. Surgeons regularly hear "I never realized how incapacitated I was until I had my pectus corrected," "I played basketball before the surgery but required frequent breaks. Now I am the fastest on my team and I can play an entire game without stopping," or similar comments.

Quality-of-life studies and overall patient satisfaction studies have shown a significant improvement in patient self-esteem and level of satisfaction after the minimally invasive repair.[8,15,34–36]

BAR REMOVAL

The bars should remain in the chest for 2 to 4 years after pectus repair. Most patients tolerate the bar well for 3 years and are able to participate in competitive sports with the bar in place (see

Fig. 4). There have been a few patients who have kept their bar in situ for 4 or more years without any problems. If patients grow more than 6 in (15 cm) after bar insertion and become symptomatic with lateral chest pain, they need to be evaluated to see if early bar removal is required.

Bar removal is accomplished under general anesthesia with positive pressure ventilation and 5 to 6 cm of positive end-expiratory pressure to prevent pneumothorax. Both sides of the bar should be mobilized, and the bar should be unbent using either the bar flippers or Multibenders (Biomet Microfixation, Jacksonville, FL, USA).[75,91,92] After straightening, the bar is removed slowly while monitoring the ECG and all the other vital signs. A postoperative chest radiograph is obtained routinely to check for pneumothorax. The complication rate for bar removal in 815 patients was 3 pneumothoraxes requiring aspiration and 1 wound infection. Elsewhere, there have been isolated reports of major complications, including 1 cardiac arrest and a pulmonary hemorrhage requiring thoracotomy.[90,93]

SUMMARY

In the 22 years since the first minimally invasive PE repair was performed, numerous modifications have made the procedure safer and more successful. As a result, there has been a dramatic increase in the number of patients seeking surgical correction. Recent studies have confirmed a reduction in the complication rate after the early learning experience, an improvement in excellent results, and a 95% overall patient satisfaction rate.[12,15]

REFERENCES

1. Nuss D, Kelly RE, Croitoru DP, et al. A 10-year review of minimally invasive technique for the correction of pectus excavatum. J Pediatr Surg 1998;33:545–52.
2. Hebra A, Swoveland B, Egbert M, et al. Outcome analysis of minimally invasive repair of pectus excavatum: review of 251 cases. J Pediatr Surg 2001; 35(2):252–8.
3. Miller KA, Woods RK, Sharp RJ, et al. Minimally invasive repair of pectus excavatum: a single institution's experience. Surgery 2001;130(4):652–7.
4. Hosie S, Sitkiewicz T, Petersen C, et al. Minimally invasive repair of pectus excavatum–the Nuss procedure. A European multicentre experience. Eur J Pediatr Surg 2002;12:235–8.
5. Uemura S, Choda Y. Nuss procedure for pectus excavatum and the operative results. Jpn J Pediatr Surg 2003;35(6):665–71.
6. Park HJ, Lee SY, Lee CS, et al. The Nuss procedure for pectus excavatum: evolution of techniques and early results on 322 patients. Ann Thorac Surg 2004;77:289–95.
7. Dzielicki J, Korlacki W, Janicka I, et al. Difficulties and limitations in minimally invasive repair of pectus excavatum-6 years experience with Nuss technique. Eur J Cardiothorac Surg 2006;30(5):801–4.
8. Pilegaard HK, Licht PB. Early results following the Nuss operation for pectus excavatum – a single-institution experience of 385 patients. Interact Cardiovasc Thorac Surg 2008;7:54–7.
9. Nuss D, Kuhn A, Obermeyer R. Our approach to MIS repair of the pectus excavatum. Contemp Surg 2007;63(9):444–53.
10. Hebra A, Gauderer MW, Tagge EP, et al. A simple technique for preventing bar displacement with the Nuss repair of pectus excavatum. J Pediatr Surg 2001;36(8):1266–8.
11. Croitoru DP, Kelly RE, Goretsky MJ, et al. Experience and modification update for the minimally invasive Nuss technique for pectus excavatum repair in 303 patients. J Pediatr Surg 2002;37:437–45.
12. Nuss D. Minimally invasive surgical repair of pectus excavatum. Semin Pediatr Surg 2008;17:209–17.
13. Boehm, Roland A, Muensterer OJ, et al. Comparing minimally invasive funnel chest repair versus the conventional technique: an outcome analysis in children. Plast Reconstr Surg 2004;114(3):668–73.
14. Petersen C, Leonhart J, Duderstadt M, et al. Minimally invasive repair of pectus excavatum-shifting the paradigm. Eur J Pediatr Surg 2006;6(2):75–8.
15. Krasopoulos G, Dusmet M, Ladas G, et al. Nuss procedure improves the quality of life in young male adults with pectus excavatum deformity. Eur J Cardiothorac Surg 2006;29:1–5.
16. Coln D, Gunning T, Ramsay M, et al. Early experience with the Nuss minimally invasive correction of pectus excavatum in adults. World J Surg 2002;10:1217–21.
17. Kim DH, Hwang JJ, Lee MK, et al. Analysis of the Nuss procedure for pectus excavatum in different age groups. Ann Thorac Surg 2005;80(3):1073–7.
18. Schalamon J, Pokall S, Windhaber J, et al. Minimally invasive correction of pectus excavatum in adult patients. J Thorac Cardiovasc Surg 2006;132(3):524–9.
19. Aronson D, Bosgraaf R, Merz E, et al. Lung function after the minimal invasive pectus excavatum repair (Nuss procedure). World J Surg 2007;31(7):1518–22.
20. Goretsky MJ, Kelly RE, Croitoru D, et al. Chest wall anomalies: pectus excavatum and pectus carinatum. Adolesc Med Clin 2004;15:455–71.
21. Nuss D. Review and discussion of the complications of minimally invasive pectus excavatum repair. Eur J Pediatr Surg 2002;12:230–4.
22. Park HJ, Lee SY, Lee CS. Complications associated with the Nuss procedure: analysis of risk factors and suggested measures for prevention of complications. J Pediatr Surg 2005;39:391–5.
23. Saxena AK, Castellani C, Hollwarth M. Surgical aspects of thoracoscopy and efficacy of right thoracoscopy in minimally invasive repair of pectus excavatum. J Thorac Cardiovasc Surg 2007;133(5):1201–5.
24. Engum S, Rescorla F, West K, et al. Is the grass greener? Early results of the Nuss procedure. J Pediatr Surg 2000;35(2):246–51.
25. Banever GT, Tashjian DB, Moriarty KP, et al. The Nuss procedure: our experience from the first fifty. Pediatr Endosurg Innov Techn 2003;7:261–6.
26. Ong C, Choo K, Morreau P, et al. The learning curve in learning the curve: a review of Nuss procedure in teenagers. ANZ J Surg 2005;75:421–4.
27. Borowitz D, Cerny F, Zallen G, et al. Pulmonary function and exercise response in patients with pectus excavatum after Nuss repair. J Pediatr Surg 2004; 38(4):544–7.
28. Lawson ML, Mellins R, Tabangin M, et al. Impact of pectus excavatum on pulmonary function before and after repair with the Nuss procedure. J Pediatr Surg 2005;40:174–80.
29. Kinuya K, Ueno T, Kobayashi T, et al. Tc-99m MAA SPECT in pectus excavatum: assessment of perfusion in volume changes after correction by the Nuss procedure. Clin Nucl Med 2005;30(12):779–82.
30. Malek MH, Berger DE, Housh TJ, et al. Cardiovascular function following surgical repair of pectus excavatum: a meta-analysis. Chest 2006;130(2):506–16.
31. Coln E, Carrasco J, Coln D. Demonstrating relief of cardiac compression with the Nuss minimally invasive repair for pectus excavatum. J Pediatr Surg 2006;41(4):683–6 [discussion: 683–6].

32. Sigalet DL, Montgomery M, Harder J, et al. Long term cardiopulmonary effects of closed repair of pectus excavatum. Pediatr Surg Int 2007;23(5):493–7.

33. Kelly R, Shamberger R, Mellins R, et al. Prospective multicenter study of surgical correction of pectus excavatum: design, perioperative complications, pain, and baseline pulmonary function facilitated by internet-based data collection. J Am Coll Surg 2007;205(2):205–16.

34. Lawson M, Cash T, Akers R, et al. A pilot study of the impact of surgical repair on disease-specific quality of life among patients with pectus excavatum. J Pediatr Surg 2003;38(6):916–8.

35. Roberts J, Hayashi A, Anderson J, et al. Quality of life of patients who have undergone the Nuss procedure for pectus excavatum: preliminary findings. J Pediatr Surg 2003;38(5):779–83.

36. Metzelder ML, Kuebler J, Leonhardt J, et al. Self and parental assessment after minimally invasive repair of pectus excavatum: lasting satisfaction after bar removal. Ann Thorac Surg 2007;83(5):1844–9.

37. Kelly RE, Cash TF, Shamberger RC, et al. Surgical repair of pectus excavatum markedly improves body image and perceived ability for physical activity: multicenter study. Pediatrics 2008;122(6):1218–22.

38. Nuss D, Kelly RE. Congenital chest wall deformities. In: Ashcraft KW, Holcomb GW III, Murphy JP, editors. Pediatric surgery. 5th edition. Philadelphia: Saunders; 2010. p. 249–65, Chapter 10.

39. Waters P, Welch K, Micheli LJ, et al. Scoliosis in children with pectus excavatum and pectus carinatum. J Pediatr Orthop 1989;9:551–6.

40. Cartoski M, Kelly RE, Nuss D, et al. Classification of the dysmorphology of pectus excavatum. J Pediatr Surg 2006;41:1573–81.

41. Mueller C, Saint-Vil D, Bouchard S. Chest x-ray as a primary modality for preoperative imaging of pectus excavatum. J Pediatr Surg 2008;43:71–3.

42. Chang PY, Lai JY, Chen JC, et al. Long-term changes in bone and cartilage after Ravitch's thoracoplasty: findings from multislice computed tomography with 3-dimensional reconstruction. J Pediatr Surg 2006;41(12):1947–50.

43. Lawson ML, Barnes-Eley M, Burke BL, et al. Reliability of a standardized protocol to calculate cross-sectional chest area and severity indices to evaluate pectus excavatum. J Pediatr Surg 2006; 41:1219–25.

44. Daunt SW, Cohen JH, Miller SF. Age-related normal ranges for the Haller index in children. Pediatr Radiol 2004;34(4):326–30.

45. Kilda A, Basevicius A, Barauskas V, et al. Radiological assessment of children with pectus excavatum. Indian J Pediatr 2007;74(2):143–7.

46. Derveaux L, Ivanoff I, Rochette F, et al. Mechanism of pulmonary function changes after surgical correction for funnel chest. Eur Respir J 1988;1(9):823–5.

47. Kaguraoka H, Ohnuki T, Itaoka T, et al. Degree of severity of pectus excavatum and pulmonary function in preoperative and postoperative periods. J Thorac Cardiovasc Surg 1992;104:1483–8.

48. Morshuis W, Folgering H, Barentsz J, et al. Pulmonary function before surgery for pectus excavatum and at long-term follow-up. Chest 1994;105(6): 1646–52.

49. Weber TR. Further experience with the operative management of asphyxiating thoracic dystrophy after pectus repair. J Pediatr Surg 2005;40:173–5.

50. Shamberger RC, Welch KJ, Sanders SP. Mitral valve prolapse associated with pectus excavatum. J Pediatr 1987;111:404–7.

51. Saint-Mezard G, Duret JC, Chanudet X. Mitral valve prolapse and pectus excavatum. Presse Med 1986; 15:439.

52. Warth DC, King ME, Cohen JM. Prevalence of mitral valve prolapse in normal children. J Am Coll Cardiol 1985;5:1173–7.

53. Raggi P, Callister TQ, Lippolis NJ, et al. Is mitral valve prolapse due to cardiac entrapment in the chest cavity? A CT view. Chest 2000;117(3):636–42.

54. Nuss D, Croitoru DP, Kelly RE. Congenital chest wall deformities. In: Ashcraft KW, Holcomp GW III, Murphy JP, editors. Pediatric surgery. 4th edition. Philadelphia: Elsevier Saunders; 2005. p. 245–63.

55. Mocchegiani R, Badano L, Lestulli C, et al. Relation of right ventricular morphology and function in pectus excavatum to the severity of the chest wall deformity. Am J Cardiol 1995;76:941–6.

56. Garusi GF, D'Ettorre A. Angiocardiographic patterns in funnel-chest. Cardiologia 1964;45:312.

57. Bevegard S. Postural circulatory changes at rest and during exercise in patients with funnel chest, with special reference to factors affecting the stroke volume. Acta Med Scand 1962;171:695.

58. Beseir GD, Epstein SE, Stampfer M, et al. Impairment of cardiac function in patients with pectus excavatum, with improvement after operative correction. N Engl J Med 1972;287:267.

59. Heitzer TA, Wollschlager H. Pectus excavatum with interior ischemia in right lateral position. Circulation 1998;98:605–6.

60. Theerthakarai R, El-Halees W, Javadpoor S, et al. Severe pectus excavatum associated with cor pulmonale and chronic respiratory acidosis in a young woman. Chest 2001;119(6):1957–61.

61. Malek MH, Fonkalsrud EW, Cooper CB. Ventilatory and cardiovascular responses to exercise in patients with pectus excavatum. Chest 2003;124:870–82.

62. Rumsey N, Harcourt D. Body image and disfigurement: issues and intervention. Body Image 2004;1: 83–97.

63. Wheeler R, Foote K. Pectus excavatum: studiously ignored in the United Kingdom? Arch Dis Child 2000;82(3):187–8.

64. Moss TP. The relationships between objective and subjective ratings of disfigurement severity, and psychological adjustment. Body Image 2005;2: 151–9.

65. Ong J, Clarke A, White P, et al. Does severity predict distress? The relationship between subjective and objective measures of appearance and psychological adjustment, during treatment for facial lipoatrophy. Body Image: Int J Research 2007;4:239–48.

66. Tebble NJ, Thomas DW, Price P. Anxiety and self-consciousness in patients with minor facial lacerations. J Adv Nurs 2004;47:417–26.

67. Uemura S, Nakagawa Y, Yoshida A, et al. Experience in 100 cases with the Nuss procedure using a technique for stabilization of the pectus bar. Pediatr Surg Int 2003;19:186–9.

68. Ohno K, Morotomi Y, Ueda M, et al. Comparison of the Nuss procedure for pectus excavatum by age and uncommon complications. Osaka City Med J 2003;49(3):71–9.

69. Rushing GD, Goretsky MJ, Gustin T, et al. When it's not an infection: metal allergy after the Nuss procedure for repair of pectus excavatum. J Pediatr Surg 2007;42:93–7.

70. Milanez de Campos JR, Fonseca MH, Werebe Ede C, et al. Technical modification of the Nuss operation for the correction of pectus excavatum. Clinics (Sao Paulo) 2006;61(2):185–6.

71. Hendrickson RJ, Bensard DD, Jarick JS, et al. Efficacy of left thoracoscopy and blunt mediastinal dissection during the Nuss procedure for pectus excavatum. J Pediatr Surg 2005;40:1312–4.

72. Bufo AJ, Stone MM. Addition of thoracoscopy to Nuss pectus excavatum repair. Pediatr Endosurg Innov Techn 2001;5(2):159–62.

73. Zallen GS, Glick PL. Miniature access pectus excavatum repair: lessons we have learned. J Pediatr Surg 2004;39(5):685–9.

74. Schaarschmidt K, Kolberg-Schwerdt A, Lempe M, et al. Extrapleural submuscular bars placed by bilateral thoracoscopy – a new improvement in modified Nuss funnel chest repair. J Pediatr Surg 2005;40:1407–10.

75. Palmer B, Yedlin S, Kim S, et al. Decreased risk of complications with bilateral thoracoscopy and left-to-right mediastinal dissection during minimally invasive repair of pectus excavatum. Eur J Pediatr Surg 2007;17:81–3.

76. Furukawa H, Sasaki S, William M, et al. Modification of thoracoscopy in pectus excavatum: insertion of both thoracoscope and introducer through a single incision to maximize visualization. Scand J Plast Surg Hand Surg 2007;41:189–92.

77. Schier F, Bahr M, Klobe E, et al. The vacuum chest wall lifter: an innovative, non-surgical addition to the management of pectus excavatum. J Pediatr Surg 2005;40:496–500.

78. Jacobs J, Quintessenza J, Morell V, et al. Minimally invasive endoscopic repair of pectus excavatum. Eur J Cardiothorac Surg 2002;21:869–73.

79. Croitoru D, Kelly R Jr, Goretsky M, et al. The minimally invasive Nuss technique for recurrent or failed pectus excavatum repair in 50 patients. J Pediatr Surg 2005;40:1.

80. Metzelder M, Ure B, Leonhardt J, et al. Impact of concomitant thoracic interventions on feasibility of Nuss procedure. J Pediatr Surg 2007;42: 1853–9.

81. Shin S, Goretsky MJ, Kelly RE Jr, et al. Infectious complications after the Nuss repair in a series of 863 patients. J Pediatr Surg 2007;42:87–92.

82. Van Renterghem KM, von Bismarck S, Bax N, et al. Should an infected Nuss bar be removed? J Pediatr Surg 2005;40:670–3.

83. Calkins CM, Shew S, Sharp R, et al. Management of postoperative infections after the minimally invasive pectus repair. J Pediatr Surg 2005;40:1004–8.

84. Watanabe A, Watanabe T, Obama T, et al. The use of a lateral stabilizer increases the incidence of wound trouble following the procedure. Ann Thorac Surg 2004;77:296–300.

85. Saitoh C, Yamada A, Kosaka K, et al. Allergy to pectus bar for funnel chest. Plast Reconstr Surg 2002; 110(2):719–21.

86. Muensterer OJ, Schenk D, Praun M, et al. Postpericardiotomy syndrome after minimally invasive pectus excavatum repair unresponsive to non-steroidal anti-inflammatory treatment. Eur J Pediatr Surg 2003;13:206–8.

87. Nuss D, Kelly REJR, Couitoru D, et al. Repair of pectus excavatum. Pediatr Endosurg Innov Techn 1999; 2(4):205–21.

88. Zoeller G. Cardiopulmonary resuscitation in patients with a Nuss bar – a case report and review of the literature. J Pediatr Surg 2005;40(11):1788–91.

89. Moss R, Albanese CT, Reynolds M. Major complications after minimally invasive repair of pectus excavatum: case reports. J Pediatr Surg 2001;36: 155–8.

90. Bouchard S, Hong AR, Gilchrist BF, et al. Catastrophic cardiac injuries encountered during the minimally invasive repair of pectus excavatum. Semin Pediatr Surg 2009;18(2):66–72.

91. Noguchi M, Fujita K. A new technique for removing the pectus bar used in the Nuss procedure. J Pediatr Surg 2005;40:674–7.

92. St Peter SD, Sharp R, Upadhyaya P, et al. A straightforward technique for removal of the substernal bar after the Nuss operation. J Pediatr Surg 2007;42:1789–91.

93. Leonhardt J, Kubler J, Feiter J, et al. Complications of the minimally invasive repair of pectus excavatum. J Pediatr Surg 2005;40(1):e7–9.

Index

Note: Page numbers of article titles are in **boldface** type.

Thorac Surg Clin 20 (2010) 599–604
doi:10.1016/S1547-4127(10)00151-9
1547-4127/10/$ – see front matter © 2010 Elsevier Inc. All rights reserved.

thoracic.theclinics.com

United States Postal Service

Statement of Ownership, Management, and Circulation
(All Periodicals Publications Except Requestor Publications)

1. Publication Title	2. Publication Number									3. Filing Date
Thoracic Surgery Clinics	0	1	3	-	1	2	6			9/15/10

4. Issue Frequency	5. Number of Issues Published Annually	6. Annual Subscription Price
Feb, May, Aug, Nov	4	$269.00

7. Complete Mailing Address of Known Office of Publication *(Not printer) (Street, city, county, state, and ZIP+4®)*

Elsevier Inc.
360 Park Avenue South
New York, NY 10010-1710

Contact Person
Stephen Bushing
Telephone *(Include area code)*
215-239-3688

8. Complete Mailing Address of Headquarters or General Business Office of Publisher *(Not printer)*

Elsevier Inc., 360 Park Avenue South, New York, NY 10010-1710

9. Full Names and Complete Mailing Addresses of Publisher, Editor, and Managing Editor *(Do not leave blank)*

Publisher *(Name and complete mailing address)*

Kim Murphy, Elsevier, Inc., 1600 John F. Kennedy Blvd. Suite 1800, Philadelphia, PA 19103-2899

Editor *(Name and complete mailing address)*

Catherine Bewick, Elsevier, Inc., 1600 John F. Kennedy Blvd. Suite 1800, Philadelphia, PA 19103-2899

Managing Editor *(Name and complete mailing address)*

Catherine Bewick, Elsevier, Inc., 1600 John F. Kennedy Blvd. Suite 1800, Philadelphia, PA 19103-2899

10. Owner *(Do not leave blank. If the publication is owned by a corporation, give the name and address of the corporation immediately followed by the names and addresses of all stockholders owning or holding 1 percent or more of the total amount of stock. If not owned by a corporation, give the names and addresses of the individual owners. If owned by a partnership or other unincorporated firm, give its name and address as well as those of each individual owner. If the publication is published by a nonprofit organization, give its name and address.)*

Full Name	Complete Mailing Address
Wholly owned subsidiary of	4520 East-West Highway
Reed/Elsevier, US holdings	Bethesda, MD 20814

11. Known Bondholders, Mortgagees, and Other Security Holders Owning or Holding 1 Percent or More of Total Amount of Bonds, Mortgages, or Other Securities. If none, check box → ☐ None

Full Name	Complete Mailing Address
N/A	

12. Tax Status *(For completion by nonprofit organizations authorized to mail at nonprofit rates) (Check one)*
The purpose, function, and nonprofit status of this organization and the exempt status for federal income tax purposes:
☒ Has Not Changed During Preceding 12 Months
☐ Has Changed During Preceding 12 Months *(Publisher must submit explanation of change with this statement)*

PS Form 3526, September 2007 (Page 1 of 3 (Instructions Page 3)) PSN 7530-01-000-9931 PRIVACY NOTICE: See our Privacy policy in www.usps.com

---

13. Publication Title		14. Issue Date for Circulation Data Below
Thoracic Surgery Clinics		August 2010

15. Extent and Nature of Circulation			14. Average No. Copies Each Issue During Preceding 12 Months	No. Copies of Single Issue Published Nearest to Filing Date
a. Total Number of Copies *(Net press run)*			1316	1291
b. Paid Circulation (By Mail and Outside the Mail)	(1)	Mailed Outside-County Paid Subscriptions Stated on PS Form 3541 *(Include paid distribution above nominal rate, advertiser's proof copies, and exchange copies)*	613	561
	(2)	Mailed In-County Paid Subscriptions Stated on PS Form 3541 *(Include paid distribution above nominal rate, advertiser's proof copies, and exchange copies)*		
	(3)	Paid Distribution Outside the Mails Including Sales Through Dealers and Carriers, Street Vendors, Counter Sales, and Other Paid Distribution Outside USPS®	275	255
	(4)	Paid Distribution by Other Classes Mailed Through the USPS *(e.g. First-Class Mail®)*		
c. Total Paid Distribution *(Sum of 15b (1), (2), (3), and (4))* ▶			888	816
d. Free or Nominal Rate Distribution (By Mail and Outside the Mail)	(1)	Free or Nominal Rate Outside-County Copies Included on PS Form 3541	40	26
	(2)	Free or Nominal Rate In-County Copies Included on PS Form 3541		
	(3)	Free or Nominal Rate Copies Mailed at Other Classes Through the USPS (e.g. First-Class Mail)		
	(4)	Free or Nominal Rate Distribution Outside the Mail *(Carriers or other means)*		
e. Total Free or Nominal Rate Distribution *(Sum of 15d (1), (2), (3) and (4))* ▶			40	26
f. Total Distribution *(Sum of 15c and 15e)* ▶			928	842
g. Copies not Distributed *(See instructions to publishers #4 (page #3))* ▶			388	449
h. Total *(Sum of 15f and g)* ▶			1316	1291
i. Percent Paid *(15c divided by 15f times 100)*			95.69%	96.91%

16. Publication of Statement of Ownership

If the publication is a general publication, publication of this statement is required. Will be printed in the November 2010 issue of this publication. ☐ Publication not required.

17. Signature and Title of Editor, Publisher, Business Manager, or Owner

Stephen R. Bushing — Fulfillment/Inventory Specialist

Date September 15, 2010

I certify that all information furnished on this form is true and complete. I understand that anyone who furnishes false or misleading information on this form or who omits material or information requested on the form may be subject to criminal sanctions (including fines and imprisonment) and/or civil sanctions (including civil penalties).

PS Form 3526, September 2007 (Page 2 of 3)

Moving?

Make sure your subscription moves with you!

To notify us of your new address, find your **Clinics Account Number** (located on your mailing label above your name), and contact customer service at:

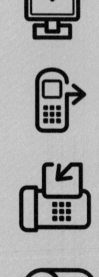

Email: journalscustomerservice-usa@elsevier.com

800-654-2452 (subscribers in the U.S. & Canada)
314-447-8871 (subscribers outside of the U.S. & Canada)

Fax number: 314-447-8029

Elsevier Health Sciences Division
Subscription Customer Service
3251 Riverport Lane
Maryland Heights, MO 63043

*To ensure uninterrupted delivery of your subscription, please notify us at least 4 weeks in advance of move.

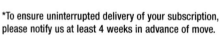

Printed and bound by CPI Group (UK) Ltd, Croydon, CR0 4YY

03/10/2024

01040351-0019